eMedguides™
.com

online and in-print Internet directories in medicine

a patient guide to

Epilepsy

resources on the **Internet**

Consulting Editor

Gregory K. Bergey, M.D.

Director, The Johns Hopkins Epilepsy Center
Professor of Neurology
The Johns Hopkins University School of Medicine

Visit **Epilepsy**
at www.eMedguides.com

eMedguides.com, Inc., a Thomson Healthcare company, Princeton, New Jersey

About the Editor:
Gregory K. Bergey, M.D.

Dr. Bergey is a Professor of Neurology at The Johns Hopkins University School of Medicine in Baltimore, Maryland, and Director of The Johns Hopkins Epilepsy Center. He was the former President of the Epilepsy Association of Maryland and is currently a member of the Board of Directors of the American Epilepsy Society and Chairman of the Advisory Board for the National EpiFellows Foundation. Dr. Bergey has published numerous book chapters and papers on a variety of aspects of epilepsy, and serves as Associate Editor of *Epilepsy Currents* and on the editorial board of *Epilepsia*.

© 2002 eMedguides.com, Inc.
eMedguides.com, Inc.
Princeton, NJ 08540

For electronic browsing of this book, see http://www.eMedguides.com/epilepsy

Sales Department
eMedguides.com, Inc.
15 Roszel Road
Princeton, NJ 08540
tel   800-230-1481 x16
fax   609-520-2023
e-mail sales@eMedguides.com
web   http://www.eMedguides.com/books

This book is set in Avenir, BaseNine, Gill Sans, and Sabon typefaces and was printed and bound in the United States of America.

10 9 8 7 6 5 4 3 2 1

ISBN 0-9716450-7-8

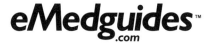

A Patient Guide to Epilepsy Resources on the Internet

Consulting Editor:
Gregory K. Bergey, M.D.
Director, The Johns Hopkins Epilepsy Center
Professor of Neurology
The Johns Hopkins University School of Medicine

Publisher:
Daniel R. Goldenson

Managing Editor:
Karen B. Schwartz

Production Editor:
Ravpreet S. Syalee

eMedguides.com, Inc., a Thomson Healthcare company

15 Roszel Road, Princeton, NJ 08540

Daniel R. Goldenson, *General Manager*

Amy Ma, Ph.D., *Coordinator,*
Publication Development

Kim Seok, *Coordinator,*
Finance Administration

Book Orders & Feedback

Book orders • http://www.eMedguides.com/books
Phone orders • 800.230.1481 x16
Facsimile • 609.520.2023
E-mail • epilepsy@eMedguides.com
Web • http://www.eMedguides.com/epilepsy

Disclaimer

eMedguides.com, Inc., hereafter referred to as the "publisher," has developed this book for informational purposes only, and not as a source of medical advice. The publisher does not guarantee the accuracy, adequacy, timeliness, or completeness of any information in this book and is not responsible for any errors or omissions or any consequences arising from the use of the information contained in this book. The material provided is general in nature and is in summary form. The content of this book is not intended in any way to be a substitute for professional medical advice. One should always seek the advice of a physician or other qualified healthcare provider. Further, one should never disregard medical advice or delay in seeking it because of information found through an Internet Web site included in this book. The use of the eMedguides.com, Inc. book is at the reader's own risk.

All information contained in this book is subject to change. Mention of a specific product, company, organization, Web site URL address, treatment, therapy, or any other topic does not imply a recommendation or endorsement by the publisher.

Non-liability

The publisher does not assume any liability for the contents of this book or the contents of any material provided at the Internet sites, companies, and organizations reviewed in this book. Moreover, the publisher assumes no liability or responsibility for damage or injury to persons or property arising from the publication and use of this book; the use of those products, services, information, ideas, or instructions contained in the material provided at the third-party Internet Web sites, companies, and organizations listed in this book; or any loss of profit or commercial damage including but not limited to special, incidental, consequential, or any other damages in connection with or arising out of the publication and use of this book. Use of third-party Web sites is subject to the Terms and Conditions of use for such sites.

Copyright Protection

Information available over the Internet and other online locations may be subject to copyright and other rights owned by third parties. Online availability of text and images does not imply that they may be reused without the permission of rights holders. Care should be taken to ensure that all necessary rights are cleared prior to reusing material distributed over the Internet and other online locations.

Trademark Protection

The words in this book for which we have reason to believe trademark, service mark, or other proprietary rights may exist have been designated as such by use of initial capitalization. However, no attempt has been made to designate as trademarks or service marks all personal computer words or terms in which proprietary rights might exist. The inclusion, exclusion, or definition of a word or term is not intended to affect, or to express any judgment on, the validity or legal status of any proprietary right that may be claimed in that word or term.

TABLE OF CONTENTS

1

INTRODUCTION

Epilepsy is defined as recurrent seizures or the tendency to have recurrent seizures. More than two million people in the United States, almost 1 percent of the entire population, have epilepsy. Another term for epilepsy is seizure disorder. Many people, perhaps 10 percent of the population, may have a single seizure during their lifetime. This is often not epilepsy. Seizures caused by metabolic causes (e.g. low blood sugar), drugs or alcohol, are not epilepsy. Epilepsy is a complex condition because of the many causes, forms, and degrees of severity. Seizure disorders can affect all ages, from the very young to the very old.

This booklet, underwritten by an unrestricted educational grant from Ortho-McNeil, a division of Johnson & Johnson, offers a thorough discussion of every facet of epilepsy, along with extensive Internet resources for further education and personal research.

Today, individuals and their families want to know as much as they can about medical conditions that concern them. Rather than offering a brief description of epilepsy, the editors of this volume have included an authoritative article from the National Institute of Neurological Disorders and Stroke (NINDS), a division of the National Institutes of Health (NIH). This article is extremely informative and answers most questions about epilepsy.

To make the process of learning about epilepsy more dynamic, the booklet contains profiles of more than 60 Web sites that approach epilepsy from many points of view. Going online to learn more about this disease can be very rewarding, since the sites have been carefully selected to address many very specific topics, from current news headlines and research articles to seizure education, clinical trials, and therapies. There are also interesting sites on such subjects as driving, employment, and genetics, as well as valuable resources about support groups and legal rights.

The theme of this booklet is learning through the Internet. For this reason, we have included a detailed explanation entitled "Getting Online" that provides a step-by-step guide for the beginner who has not used the World Wide Web extensively. Although one must use a computer to get online, almost every library in the United States has computers available for patrons, as well as librarians willing to give a few pointers on getting started, so it is certainly not necessary to own a computer to get the most out of this booklet.

This booklet is also available on the eMedguides Web site, where the entire volume can be viewed online. The Web address to view this book is http://www.eMedguides.com/epilepsy.

We hope the readers of this special booklet will realize the potential of the Internet as a new and exciting research and education tool in the field of medicine, and will increase their knowledge not only of epilepsy but also of other health and medical topics.

— The Editors

GETTING ONLINE

The Internet is growing at a rapid pace, but many individuals are not yet online. What is preventing people from jumping on the "information highway"? There are many factors, but the most common issue is a general confusion about what the Internet is, how it works, and how to access it.

The following few pages are designed to clear up any confusion for readers who have not yet accessed the Internet. We will look at the process of getting onto and using the Internet, step by step.

It is also helpful to consult other resources, such as the technical support department of the manufacturer or store where you bought your computer. Although assistance varies widely, most organizations provide startup assistance for new users and are experienced with guiding individuals onto the Internet. Books can also be of great assistance, as they provide a simple and clear view of how computers and the Internet work, and can be studied at your own pace.

What is the Internet?

The Internet is a large network of computers that are all connected to one another. A good analogy is to envision a neighborhood, with houses and storefronts, all connected to one another by streets and highways. Often the Internet is referred to as the "information superhighway" because of the vastness of this neighborhood.

The Internet was initially developed to allow people to share computers, that is, share part of their "house" with others. The ability to connect to so many other computers quickly and easily made this feasible. As computers proliferated and increased in computational power, people started using the Internet for sending information quickly from one computer to another.

For example, the most popular feature of the Internet is electronic mail (e-mail). Each computer has a mailbox, and an electronic letter can be sent instantly. People also use the Internet to post bulletins, or other information, for others to see. The process of sending e-mail or viewing this information is simple. A computer and a connection to the Internet are all you need to begin.

How is an Internet connection provided?

The Internet is accessed either through a "direct" connection, which is found in businesses and educational institutions, or through a phone line. Phone line connections are the most common access method for users at home, although direct connections are becoming available for home use. There are many complex options in this area; for the new user it is simplest to use an existing phone line to experience the Internet for the first time. A dual telephone jack can be purchased at many retail stores. Connect the computer to the phone jack, and then use the provided software to connect to the Internet. Your computer will dial the number of an Internet provider and ask you for a user name and password. Keep in mind that while you are using the Internet, your phone line is tied up, and callers will hear a busy signal. Also, call waiting can sometimes interrupt an Internet connection and disconnect you from the Internet.

Who provides an Internet connection?

There are many providers at both the local and national levels. One of the easiest ways to get online is with America Online (AOL). They provide software and a user-friendly environment through which to access the Internet. Because AOL manages both this environment and the actual connection, they can be of great assistance when you are starting out. America Online takes you to a menu of choices when you log in, and while using their software you can read and send e-mail, view Web pages, and chat with others.

Many other similar services exist, and most of them also provide an environment using Microsoft or Netscape products. These companies, such as the Microsoft Network (MSN) and Earthlink, also provide simple, easy-to-use access to the Internet. Their environment is more standard and not limited to the choices America Online provides.

Internet connections generally run from $10-$30 per month (depending on the length of commitment) in addition to telephone costs. Most national providers have local phone numbers all over the country that should eliminate any telephone charges. The monthly provider fee is the only direct charge for accessing the Internet.

How do I get on the Internet?

Once you've signed up with an Internet provider and installed their software (often only a matter of answering basic questions), your computer will be set up to access the Internet. By double-clicking on an icon, your computer will dial the phone number, log you in, and present you with a Web page (a "home" page).

What are some of the Internet's features?

From the initial Web page there are almost limitless possibilities of where you can go. The address at the top of the screen (identified by an "http://" in front) tells you where you are. You can also type the address of where you would like to go next. When typing a new address, you do not need to add the "http://". The computer adds this prefix automatically after you type in an address and press return. Once you press return, the Web site will appear in the browser window.

You can also navigate the Web by "surfing" from one site to another using links on a page. A Web page might say, "Click here for weather." If you move the mouse pointer to this underlined phrase and click the mouse button, you will be taken to a different address, where weather information is provided.

The Internet has several other useful features. E-mail is an extremely popular and important service. It is free and messages are delivered instantly. Although you can access e-mail through a Web browser (AOL has this feature), many Internet services provide a separate e-mail program for reading, writing, and organizing your correspondence. These programs send and retrieve messages from the Internet.

Another area of the Internet offers chat rooms where users can hold roundtable discussions. In a chat room you can type messages and see the replies of other users around the world. There are chat rooms on virtually every topic, although the dialog certainly varies in this free-for-all forum. There are also newsgroups on the Internet, some of which we list in this book. A newsgroup is similar to a chat room but each message is a separate item and can be viewed in sequence at any time. For example, a user might post a question about Lyme disease. In the newsgroup you can read the question and then read the answers that others have provided. You can also post your own comments. This forum is usually not managed or edited, particularly in the medical field. Do not take the advice of a chat room or newsgroup source without first consulting your physician.

How can I find things on the Internet?
Surfing the Internet, from site to site, is a popular activity. But if you have a focused mission, you will want to use a search engine. A search engine can scan lists of Web sites to look for a particular site. We provide a long list of medical search engines in this book.

Because the Internet is so large and unregulated, sites are often hard to find. In the physical world it is difficult to find good services, but you can turn to the yellow pages or other resources to get a comprehensive list. Physical proximity is also a major factor. On the Internet, the whole world is at your doorstep. Finding a reliable site takes time and patience, and can require sifting through hundreds of similar, yet irrelevant, sites.

The most common way to find information on the Internet is to use a search engine. When you go to the Web page of a search engine, you will be presented with two distinct methods of searching: using links to topics, or using a keyword search. The links often represent the Web site staff's best effort to find quality sites. This method of searching is the core of the Yahoo! search engine (http://www.yahoo.com). By clicking on Healthcare, then Disorders, then Lung Cancer, you are provided with a list of sites the staff has found on the topic.

The keyword approach is definitely more daring. By typing in search terms, the engine looks through its list of Web sites for a match and returns the results. These engines typically only cover 15 percent of the Internet, so it is not a comprehensive process. They also usually return far too many choices. Typing lung cancer into a search engine box will return thousands of sites, including one entry for every site where someone used the words lung cancer on a personal Web page.

Where do eMedguides come in?

eMedguides are organized listings of Web sites in each major medical specialty. Our team of editors continually scours the Net, searching for quality Web sites that relate to specific specialties, disorders, and research topics. More importantly, of the sites we find, we only include those that provide professional and useful content. eMedguides fill a critical gap in the Internet research process. Each guide provides more than 1,000 Web sites that focus on every aspect of a single medical discipline.

Other Internet search engines rely on teams of "surfers" who can only cover a subject on its surface because they survey the entire Internet. Search engines, even medical search engines, return far too many choices, requiring hours of time and patience to sift through. eMedguides, on the other hand, focus on medical and physician sites in a specialty. With an eMedguide in hand, you can quickly identify the sites worth visiting on the Internet and jump right to them. At our site, http://www.eMedguides.com, you can access the same listings as in this book and can simply click on a site to go straight to it. In addition, we provide continual updates to the book through the site and annually in print. Our editors do the surfing for you and do it professionally, making your Internet experience efficient and fulfilling.

Our new e-Link identification code is the fastest way to surf the Internet. Simply append the code number to the eMedguides address (http://www.eMedguides. com/b-0101) to be taken directly to the site you are reading about in the book.

Taking medical action must involve a physician

As interesting as the Internet is, the information that you will find is both objective and subjective. Our goal is to expose our readers to Web sites on hundreds of topics for informational purposes only. If you are not a physician and become interested in the ideas, guidelines, recommendations, or experiences discussed online, bring these findings to a physician for personal evaluation. Medical needs vary considerably, and a medical approach or therapy for one individual could be entirely misguided for another. Final medical advice and a plan of action must come only from a physician.

3

Understanding Epilepsy

This article was prepared by the
National Institute of Neurological
Disorders and Stroke, Bethesda, Maryland.

3.1 Introduction

Few experiences match the drama of a convulsive seizure. A person having a severe seizure may cry out, fall to the floor unconscious, twitch or move uncontrollably, drool, or even lose bladder control. Within minutes, the attack is over, and the person regains consciousness but is exhausted and dazed. This is the image most people have when they hear the word epilepsy. However, this type of seizure—a generalized tonic-clonic seizure—is only one kind of epilepsy. There are many other kinds, each with a different set of symptoms.

Epilepsy was one of the first brain disorders to be described. It was mentioned in ancient Babylon more than 3,000 years ago. The strange behavior caused by some seizures has contributed through the ages to many superstitions and prejudices. The word epilepsy is derived from the Greek word for "attack." People once thought that those with epilepsy were being visited by demons or gods. However, in 400 B.C., the early physician Hippocrates suggested that epilepsy was a disorder of the brain—and we now know that he was right.

3.2 What is Epilepsy?

Epilepsy is a brain disorder in which clusters of nerve cells, or neurons, in the brain sometimes signal abnormally. Neurons normally generate electrochemical impulses that act on other neurons, glands, and muscles to produce human thoughts, feelings, and actions. In epilepsy, the normal pattern of neuronal activity becomes disturbed, causing strange sensations, emotions, and behavior, or sometimes *convulsions,* muscle spasms, and loss of consciousness. During a seizure, neurons may fire as many as 500 times a second, much faster than the normal rate of about 80 times a second. In some people, this happens only occasionally; for others, it may happen up to hundreds of times a day.

More than 2 million people in the United States—about 1 in 100—have experienced an unprovoked seizure or been diagnosed with epilepsy. For about 80 percent of those diagnosed with epilepsy, seizures can be controlled with modern medicines and surgical techniques. However, about 20 percent of people with epilepsy will continue to experience seizures even with the best available treatment. Doctors call this situation *intractable epilepsy*. Having a seizure does not necessarily mean that a person has epilepsy. Only when a person has had two or more seizures is he or she considered to have epilepsy.

Epilepsy is not contagious and is not caused by mental illness or mental retardation. Some people with mental retardation may experience seizures, but seizures do not necessarily mean the person has or will develop mental impairment. Many people with epilepsy have normal or above-average intelligence. Famous people who are known or rumored to have had epilepsy include the Russian writer Dostoyevsky, the philosopher Socrates, the military general Napoleon, and the inventor of dynamite, Alfred Nobel, who established the Nobel prize. Several Olympic medalists and other athletes also have had epilepsy. Seizures sometimes do cause brain damage, particularly if they are severe. However, most seizures do not seem to have a detrimental effect on the brain. Any changes that do occur are usually subtle, and it is often unclear whether these changes are caused by the seizures themselves or by the underlying problem that caused the seizures.

While epilepsy cannot currently be cured, for some people it does eventually go away. One study found that children with *idiopathic epilepsy*, or epilepsy with an unknown cause, had a 68 to 92 percent chance of becoming seizure-free by 20 years after their diagnosis. The odds of becoming seizure-free are not as good for adults, or for children with severe epilepsy syndromes, but it is nonetheless possible that seizures may decrease or even stop over time. This is more likely if the epilepsy has been well-controlled by medication or if the person has had epilepsy surgery.

3.3 WHAT CAUSES EPILEPSY?

Epilepsy is a disorder with many possible causes. Anything that disturbs the normal pattern of neuron activity—from illness to brain damage to abnormal brain development—can lead to seizures.

Epilepsy may develop because of an abnormality in brain wiring, an imbalance of nerve signaling chemicals called *neurotransmitters*, or some combination of these factors. Researchers believe that some people with epilepsy have an abnormally high level of *excitatory neurotransmitters* that increase neuronal activity, while others have an abnormally low level of *inhibitory neurotransmitters* that decrease neuronal activity in the brain. Either situation can result in too much neuronal activity and cause epilepsy. One of the most-studied neurotransmitters that plays a role in epilepsy is *GABA*, or gamma-aminobutyric acid, which is an inhibitory neurotransmitter. Research on GABA has led to drugs that alter the amount of this neurotransmitter in the brain or change how the brain responds to it. Researchers also are studying excitatory neurotransmitters such as *glutamate*.

In some cases, the brain's attempts to repair itself after a head injury, stroke, or other problem may inadvertently generate abnormal nerve connections that lead to epilepsy. Abnormalities in brain wiring that occur during brain development also may disturb neuronal activity and lead to epilepsy.

Research has shown that the cell membrane that surrounds each neuron plays an important role in epilepsy. Cell membranes are crucial for neurons to generate electrical impulses. For this reason, researchers are studying details of the membrane structure, how molecules move in and out of membranes, and how the cell nourishes and repairs the membrane. A disruption in any of these processes may lead to epilepsy. Studies in animals have shown that, because the brain continually adapts to changes in stimuli, a small change in neuronal activity, if repeated, may eventually lead to full-blown epilepsy. Researchers are investigating whether this phenomenon, called *kindling,* may also occur in humans.

In some cases, epilepsy may result from changes in non-neuronal brain cells called glia. These cells regulate concentrations of chemicals in the brain that can affect neuronal signaling.

About half of all seizures have no known cause. However, in other cases, the seizures are clearly linked to infection, trauma, or other identifiable problems.

GENETIC FACTORS

Research suggests that genetic abnormalities may be some of the most important factors contributing to epilepsy. Some types of epilepsy have been traced to an abnormality in a specific gene. Many other types of epilepsy tend to run in families, which suggests that genes influence epilepsy. Some researchers estimate that more than 500 genes could play a role in this disorder. However, it is increasingly clear that, for many forms of epilepsy, genetic abnormalities play only a partial role, perhaps by increasing a person's susceptibility to seizures that are triggered by an environmental factor.

Several types of epilepsy have now been linked to defective genes for *ion channels,* the "gates" that control the flow of *ions* in and out of cells and regulate neuron signaling. Another gene, which is missing in people with *progressive myoclonus epilepsy,* codes for a protein called cystatin B. This protein regulates enzymes that break down other proteins. Another gene, which is altered in a severe form of epilepsy called *LaFora's disease,* has been linked to a gene that helps to break down carbohydrates.

While abnormal genes sometimes cause epilepsy, they also may influence the disorder in subtler ways. For example, one study showed that many people with epilepsy have an abnormally active version of a gene that increases resistance to drugs. This may help explain why anticonvulsant drugs do not work for some people. Genes also may control other aspects of the body's response to medications and each person's susceptibility to seizures, or *seizure threshold*. Abnormalities in the genes that control neuronal migration—a critical step in brain development—can lead to areas of misplaced or abnormally formed neurons, or *dysplasia*, in the brain that can cause epilepsy. In some cases, genes may contribute to development of epilepsy even in people with no family history of the disorder. These people may have a newly developed abnormality, or *mutation*, in an epilepsy-related gene.

OTHER DISORDERS

In many cases, epilepsy develops as a result of brain damage from other disorders. For example, brain tumors, alcoholism, and Alzheimer's disease frequently lead to epilepsy because they alter the normal workings of the brain. Strokes, heart attacks, and other conditions that deprive the brain of oxygen also can cause epilepsy in some cases. About 32 percent of all newly developed epilepsy in elderly people appears to be due to cerebrovascular disease, which reduces the supply of oxygen to brain cells. Meningitis, AIDS, viral encephalitis, and other infectious diseases can lead to epilepsy, as can hydrocephalus—a condition in which excess fluid builds up in the brain. Epilepsy also can result from intolerance to wheat gluten (known as *celiac* disease), or from a parasitic infection of the brain called *neurocysticercosis*. Seizures may stop once these disorders are treated successfully. However, the odds of becoming seizure-free after the primary disorder is treated are uncertain and vary depending on the type of disorder, the brain region that is affected, and how much brain damage occurred prior to treatment.

Epilepsy is associated with a variety of developmental and metabolic disorders, including cerebral palsy, neurofibromatosis, pyruvate deficiency, tuberous sclerosis, Landau-Kleffner syndrome, and autism. Epilepsy is just one of a set of symptoms commonly found in people with these disorders.

HEAD INJURY

In some cases, head injury can lead to seizures or epilepsy. Safety measures such as wearing seat belts in cars and using helmets when riding a motorcycle or playing competitive sports can protect people from epilepsy and other problems that result from head injury.

Prenatal Injury and Developmental Problems

The developing brain is susceptible to many kinds of injury. Maternal infections, poor nutrition, and oxygen deficiencies are just some of the conditions that may take a toll on the brain of a developing baby. These conditions may lead to cerebral palsy, which often is associated with epilepsy, or they may cause epilepsy that is unrelated to any other disorders. About 20 percent of seizures in children are due to cerebral palsy or other neurological abnormalities. Abnormalities in genes that control development also may contribute to epilepsy. Advanced brain imaging has revealed that some cases of epilepsy that occur with no obvious cause may be associated with areas of dysplasia in the brain that probably develop before birth.

Poisoning

Seizures can result from exposure to lead, carbon monoxide, and many other poisons. They also can result from exposure to street drugs and from overdoses of antidepressants and other medications.

Seizures are often triggered by factors such as lack of sleep, alcohol consumption, stress, or hormonal changes associated with the menstrual cycle. These *seizure triggers* do not cause epilepsy but can provoke first seizures or cause breakthrough seizures in people who otherwise experience good seizure control with their medication. Sleep deprivation in particular is a universal and powerful trigger of seizures. For this reason, people with epilepsy should make sure to get enough sleep and should try to stay on a regular sleep schedule as much as possible. For some people, light flashing at a certain speed or the flicker of a computer monitor can trigger a seizure; this problem is called *photosensitive epilepsy*. Smoking cigarettes also can trigger seizures. The nicotine in cigarettes acts on receptors for the excitatory neurotransmitter acetylcholine in the brain, which increases neuronal firing. Seizures are not triggered by sexual activity except in very rare instances.

3.4 What Are the Different Kinds of Seizures?

Doctors have described more than 30 different types of seizures. Seizures are divided into two major categories—*partial seizures* and *generalized seizures*. However, there are many different types of seizures in each of these categories.

Partial Seizures

Partial seizures occur in just one part of the brain. About 60 percent of people with epilepsy have partial seizures. These seizures are frequently described by the area of the brain in which they originate. For example, someone might be diagnosed with partial frontal lobe seizures.

In a *simple partial seizure,* the person will remain conscious but may experience unusual feelings or sensations that can take many forms. The person may experience sudden and unexplainable feelings of joy, anger, sadness, or nausea. He or she also may hear, smell, taste, see, or feel things that are not real.

In a *complex partial seizure,* the person has a change in or loss of consciousness. His or her consciousness may be altered, producing a dreamlike experience. People having a complex partial seizure may display strange, repetitious behaviors such as blinks, twitches, mouth movements, or even walking in a circle. These repetitive movements are called *automatisms.* They also may fling objects across the room or strike out at walls or furniture as though they are angry or afraid. These seizures usually last just a few seconds.

Some people with partial seizures, especially complex partial seizures, may experience *auras*—unusual sensations that warn of an impending seizure. These auras are actually simple partial seizures in which the person maintains consciousness. The symptoms an individual person has, and the progression of those symptoms, tends to be *stereotyped,* or similar every time.

The symptoms of partial seizures can easily be confused with other disorders. For instance, the dreamlike perceptions associated with a complex partial seizure may be misdiagnosed as migraine headaches, which also can cause a dreamlike state. The strange behavior and sensations caused by partial seizures also can be mistaken for symptoms of narcolepsy, fainting, or even mental illness. It may take many tests and careful monitoring by a knowledgeable physician to tell the difference between epilepsy and other disorders.

GENERALIZED SEIZURES

Generalized seizures are a result of abnormal neuronal activity in many parts of the brain. These seizures may cause loss of consciousness, falls, or massive muscle spasms.

There are many kinds of generalized seizures. In *absence* seizures, the person may appear to be staring into space and/or have jerking or twitching muscles. These seizures are sometimes referred to as *petit mal seizures,* which is an older term. *Tonic seizures* cause stiffening of muscles of the body, generally those in the back, legs, and arms. *Clonic seizures* cause repeated jerking movements of muscles on both sides of the body. *Myoclonic seizures* cause jerks or twitches of the upper body, arms, or legs. *Atonic seizures* cause a loss of normal muscle tone. The affected person will fall down or may nod his or her head involuntarily. *Tonic-clonic* seizures cause a mixture of symptoms, including stiffening of the body and repeated jerks of the arms and/or legs as well as loss of consciousness. Tonic-clonic seizures are sometimes referred to by an older term: *grand mal seizures.*

Not all seizures can be easily defined as either partial or generalized. Some people have seizures that begin as partial seizures but then spread to the entire brain. Other people may have both types of seizures but with no clear pattern.

Society's lack of understanding about the many different types of seizures is one of the biggest problems for people with epilepsy. People who witness a non-convulsive seizure often find it difficult to understand that behavior which looks deliberate is not under the person's control. In some cases, this has led to the affected person being arrested, sued, or placed in a mental institution. To combat these problems, people everywhere need to understand the many different types of seizures and how they may appear.

3.5 WHAT ARE THE DIFFERENT KINDS OF EPILEPSY?

Just as there are many different kinds of seizures, there are many different kinds of epilepsy. Doctors have identified hundreds of different *epilepsy* syndromes— disorders characterized by a specific set of symptoms that include epilepsy. Some of these syndromes appear to be hereditary. For other syndromes, the cause is unknown. Epilepsy syndromes are frequently described by their symptoms or by where in the brain they originate. People should discuss the implications of their type of epilepsy with their doctors to understand the full range of symptoms, the possible treatments, and the prognosis.

People with *absence epilepsy* have repeated absence seizures that cause momentary lapses of consciousness. These seizures almost always begin in childhood or adolescence, and they tend to run in families, suggesting that they may be at least partially due to a defective gene or genes. Some people with absence seizures have purposeless movements during their seizures, such as a jerking arm or rapidly blinking eyes. Others have no noticeable symptoms except for brief times when they are "out of it." Immediately after a seizure, the person can resume whatever he or she was doing. However, these seizures may occur so frequently that the person cannot concentrate in school or other situations. Childhood absence epilepsy usually stops when the child reaches puberty. Absence seizures usually have no lasting effect on intelligence or other brain functions.

Psychomotor epilepsy

Psychomotor epilepsy is another term for recurrent partial seizures, especially seizures of the temporal lobe. The term psychomotor refers to the strange sensations, emotions, and behavior seen with these seizures.

Temporal lobe epilepsy

Temporal lobe epilepsy, or TLE, is the most common epilepsy syndrome with partial seizures. These seizures are often associated with auras. TLE often begins in childhood. Research has shown that repeated temporal lobe seizures can cause a brain structure called the *hippocampus* to shrink over time. The hippocampus is important for memory and learning. While it may take years of temporal lobe seizures for measurable hippocampal damage to occur, this finding underlines the need to treat TLE early and as effectively as possible.

Frontal lobe epilepsy

Frontal lobe epilepsy usually involves a cluster of short seizures with a sudden onset and termination. There are many subtypes of frontal lobe seizures. The symptoms depend on where in the frontal lobe the seizures occur.

Occipital lobe epilepsy

Occipital lobe epilepsy usually begins with visual hallucinations, rapid eye blinking, or other eye-related symptoms. Otherwise, it resembles temporal or frontal lobe epilepsy.

The symptoms of *parietal lobe epilepsy* closely resemble those of other types of epilepsy. This may reflect the fact that parietal lobe seizures tend to spread to other areas of the brain.

There are many other types of epilepsy, each with its own characteristic set of symptoms. Many of these, including *Lennox-Gastaut syndrome* and *Rasmussen's encephalitis*, begin in childhood. Children with Lennox-Gastaut syndrome have severe epilepsy with several different types of seizures, including atonic seizures, which cause sudden falls and are also called *drop attacks*. This severe form of epilepsy can be very difficult to treat effectively. Rasmussen's encephalitis is a progressive type of epilepsy in which half of the brain shows continual inflammation. It sometimes is treated with a radical surgical procedure called hemispherectomy (see the section on *Surgery*). Some childhood epilepsy syndromes, such as childhood absence epilepsy, tend to go into remission or stop entirely during adolescence, whereas other syndromes such as *juvenile* myoclonic epilepsy are usually present for life once they develop. Seizure syndromes do not always appear in childhood. For example, *Ramsay Hunt syndrome type II* is a rare and severe progressive type of epilepsy that generally begins in early adulthood and leads to reduced muscle coordination and cognitive abilities in addition to seizures.

Epilepsy syndromes that do not seem to impair cognitive functions or development are often described as *benign*. Benign epilepsy syndromes include *benign infantile* encephalopathy and *benign neonatal convulsions*. Other syndromes, such as *early* myoclonic encephalopathy, include neurological and developmental problems. However, these problems may be caused by underlying neurodegenerative processes rather than by the seizures. Epilepsy syndromes in which the seizures and/or the person's cognitive or motor abilities get worse over time are called *progressive epilepsy.*

Several types of epilepsy begin in infancy. The most common type of infantile epilepsy is *infantile spasms,* clusters of seizures that usually begin before the age of 6 months. During these seizures the infant may bend and cry out. Anticonvulsant drugs often do not work for infantile spasms, but the seizures can be treated with *ACTH* (adrenocorticotropic hormone) or *prednisone.*

3.6 When Are Seizures Not Epilepsy?

While any seizure is cause for concern, having a seizure does not by itself mean a person has epilepsy. First seizures, febrile seizures, nonepileptic events, and eclampsia are examples of seizures that may not be associated with epilepsy.

First Seizures

Many people have a single seizure at some point in their lives. Often these seizures occur in reaction to anesthesia or a strong drug, but they also may be unprovoked, meaning that they occur without any obvious triggering factor. Unless the person has suffered brain damage or there is a family history of epilepsy or other neurological abnormalities, these single seizures usually are not followed by additional seizures. One recent study that followed patients for an average of 8 years found that only 33 percent of people have a second seizure within 4 years after an initial seizure. People who did not have a second seizure within that time remained seizure-free for the rest of the study. For people who did have a second seizure, the risk of a third seizure was about 73 percent on average by the end of 4 years.

When someone has experienced a first seizure, the doctor will usually order an *electroencephalogram,* or *EEG,* to determine what type of seizure the person may have had and if there are any detectable abnormalities in the person's brain waves. The doctor also may order brain scans to identify abnormalities that may be visible in the brain. These tests may help the doctor decide whether or not to treat the person with antiepileptic drugs. In some cases, drug treatment after the first seizure may help prevent future seizures and epilepsy. However, the drugs also can cause detrimental side effects, so doctors prescribe them only when they feel the benefits outweigh the risks. Evidence suggests that it may be beneficial to begin anticonvulsant medication once a person has had a second seizure, as the chance of future seizures increases significantly after this occurs.

FEBRILE SEIZURES

Sometimes a child will have a seizure during the course of an illness with a high fever. These seizures are called *febrile seizures* (*febrile* is derived from the Latin word for "fever") and can be very alarming to the parents and other caregivers. In the past, doctors usually prescribed a course of anticonvulsant drugs following a febrile seizure in the hope of preventing epilepsy. However, most children who have a febrile seizure do not develop epilepsy, and long-term use of anticonvulsant drugs in children may damage the developing brain or cause other detrimental side effects. Experts at a 1980 consensus conference coordinated by the National Institutes of Health concluded that preventive treatment after a febrile seizure is generally not warranted unless certain other conditions are present: a family history of epilepsy, signs of nervous system impairment prior to the seizure, or a relatively prolonged or complicated seizure. The risk of subsequent non-febrile seizures is only 2 to 3 percent unless one of these factors is present.

Researchers have now identified several different genes that influence the risk of febrile seizures in certain families. Studying these genes may lead to new understanding of how febrile seizures occur and perhaps point to ways of preventing them.

NONEPILEPTIC EVENTS

Sometimes people appear to have seizures, even though their brains show no seizure activity. This type of phenomenon has various names, including nonepileptic events and pseudoseizures. Both of these terms essentially mean something that looks like a seizure but isn't one. Nonepileptic events that are psychological in origin may be referred to as psychogenic seizures. Psychogenic seizures may indicate dependence, a need for attention, avoidance of stressful situations, or specific psychiatric conditions. Some people with epilepsy have psychogenic seizures in addition to their epileptic seizures. Other people who have psychogenic seizures do not have epilepsy at all. Psychogenic seizures cannot be treated in the same way as epileptic seizures. Instead, they are often treated by mental health specialists.

Other nonepileptic events may be caused by narcolepsy, Tourette syndrome, cardiac arrhythmia, and other medical conditions with symptoms that resemble seizures. Because symptoms of these disorders can look very much like epileptic seizures, they are often mistaken for epilepsy. Distinguishing between true epileptic seizures and nonepileptic events can be very difficult and requires a thorough medical assessment, careful monitoring, and knowledgeable health professionals. Improvements in brain scanning and monitoring technology may improve diagnosis of nonepileptic events in the future.

Eclampsia

Eclampsia is a life-threatening condition that can develop in pregnant women. Its symptoms include sudden elevations of blood pressure and seizures. Pregnant women who develop unexpected seizures should be rushed to a hospital immediately. Eclampsia can be treated in a hospital setting and usually does not result in additional seizures or epilepsy once the pregnancy is over.

3.7 How is Epilepsy Diagnosed?

Doctors have developed a number of different tests to determine whether a person has epilepsy and, if so, what kind of seizures the person has. In some cases, people may have symptoms that look very much like a seizure but in fact are nonepileptic events caused by other disorders. Even doctors may not be able to tell the difference between these disorders and epilepsy without close observation and intensive testing.

EEG Monitoring

An EEG records brain waves detected by electrodes placed on the scalp. This is the most common diagnostic test for epilepsy and can detect abnormalities in the brain's electrical activity. People with epilepsy frequently have changes in their normal pattern of brain waves, even when they are not experiencing a seizure. While this type of test can be very useful in diagnosing epilepsy, it is not foolproof. Some people continue to show normal brain wave patterns even after they have experienced a seizure. In other cases, the unusual brain waves are generated deep in the brain where the EEG is unable to detect them. Many people who do not have epilepsy also show some unusual brain activity on an EEG. Whenever possible, an EEG should be performed within 24 hours of a patient's first seizure. Ideally, EEGs should be performed while the patient is sleeping as well as when he or she is awake, because brain activity during sleep is often quite different than at other times.

Video monitoring is often used in conjunction with EEG to determine the nature of a person's seizures. It also can be used in some cases to rule out other disorders such as cardiac arrhythmia or narcolepsy that may look like epilepsy.

In some cases, doctors may use an experimental diagnostic technique called a *magnetoencephalogram*, or *MEG*. MEG detects the magnetic signals generated by neurons to allow doctors to monitor brain activity at different points in the brain over time, revealing different brain functions. While MEG is similar in concept to EEG, it does not require electrodes and it can detect signals from deeper in the brain than an EEG.

Brain Scans

One of the most important ways of diagnosing epilepsy is through the use of brain scans. The most commonly used brain scans include *CT* (computed tomography), *PET* (positron emission tomography) and *MRI* (magnetic resonance imaging). CT and MRI scans reveal the structure of the brain, which can be useful for identifying brain tumors, cysts, and other structural abnormalities. PET and an adapted kind of MRI called *functional* MRI (fMRI) can be used to monitor the brain's activity and detect abnormalities in how it works. *SPECT* (*single photon emission computed tomography*) is a relatively new kind of brain scan that is sometimes used to locate seizure foci in the brain. Doctors also are experimenting with brain scans called *magnetic resonance* spectroscopy (*MRS*) that can detect abnormalities in the brain's biochemical processes, and with *near-infrared spectroscopy,* a technique that can detect oxygen levels in brain tissue.

Medical History

Taking a detailed medical history, including symptoms and duration of the seizures, is still one of the best methods available to determine if a person has epilepsy and what kind of seizures they have. The doctor will ask questions about the seizures and any past illnesses or other symptoms a person may have had. Since people who have suffered a seizure often do not remember what happened, caregivers' accounts of the seizure are vital to this evaluation.

Blood Tests

Doctors often take blood samples for testing, particularly when they are examining a child. These blood samples are often screened for metabolic or genetic disorders that may be associated with the seizures. They also may be used to check for underlying problems such as infections, lead poisoning, anemia, and diabetes that may be causing or triggering the seizures.

Developmental, Neurological, and Behavioral Tests

Doctors often use tests devised to measure motor abilities, behavior, and intellectual capacity as a way to determine how the epilepsy is affecting that person. These tests also can provide clues about what kind of epilepsy the person has.

3.8 Can Epilepsy be Prevented?

Many cases of epilepsy can be prevented by wearing seatbelts and bicycle helmets, putting children in car seats, and other measures that prevent head injury and other trauma. Prescribing medication after first or second seizures or febrile seizures also may help prevent epilepsy in some cases. Good prenatal care, including treatment of high blood pressure and infections during pregnancy, can prevent brain damage in the developing baby that may lead to epilepsy and other neurological problems later. Treating cardiovascular disease, high blood pressure, infections, and other disorders that can affect the brain during adulthood and aging also may prevent many cases of epilepsy. Finally, identifying the genes for many neurological disorders can provide opportunities for genetic screening and prenatal diagnosis that may ultimately prevent many cases of epilepsy.

3.9 How can Epilepsy be Treated?

Accurate diagnosis of the type of epilepsy a person has is crucial for finding an effective treatment. There are many different ways to treat epilepsy. Currently available treatments can control seizures at least some of the time in about 80 percent of people with epilepsy. However, another 20 percent—about 600,000 people with epilepsy in the United States—have intractable seizures, and another 400,000 feel they get inadequate relief from available treatments. These statistics make it clear that improved treatments are desperately needed.

Doctors who treat epilepsy come from many different fields of medicine. They include neurologists, pediatricians, pediatric neurologists, internists, and family physicians, as well as neurosurgeons and doctors called epileptologists who specialize in treating epilepsy. People who need specialized or intensive care for epilepsy may be treated at large medical centers and neurology clinics at hospitals, or by neurologists in private practice. Many epilepsy treatment centers are associated with university hospitals that perform research in addition to providing medical care.

Once epilepsy is diagnosed, it is important to begin treatment as soon as possible. Research suggests that medication and other treatments may be less successful in treating epilepsy once seizures and their consequences become established.

Medications

By far the most common approach to treating epilepsy is to prescribe antiepileptic drugs. The first effective antiepileptic drugs were bromides, introduced by an English physician named Sir Charles Locock in 1857. He noticed that bromides had a sedative effect and seemed to reduce seizures in some patients. More than 20 different antiepileptic drugs are now on the market, all with different benefits and side effects. The choice of which drug to prescribe, and at what dosage, depends on many different factors, including the type of seizures a person has, the person's lifestyle and age, how frequently the seizures occur, and, for a woman, the likelihood that she will become pregnant. People with epilepsy should follow their doctor's advice and share any concerns they may have regarding their medication.

Doctors seeing a patient with newly developed epilepsy often prescribe carbamazapine, valproate, or phenytoin first, unless the epilepsy is a type that is known to require a different kind of treatment. For absence seizures, ethosuximide is often the primary treatment. Other commonly prescribed drugs include clonazepam, phenobarbital, and primidone. In recent years, a number of new drugs have become available. These include tiagabine, lamotrigine, gabapentin, topiramate, levetiracetam, and felbamate, as well as oxcarbazapine, a drug that is similar to carbamazapine but has fewer side effects. These new drugs may have advantages for many patients. Other drugs are used in combination with one of the standard drugs or for intractable seizures that do not respond to other medications. A few drugs, such as fosphenytoin, are approved for use only in hospital settings to treat specific problems such as *status epilepticus* (see section, "Are There Special Risks Associated With Epilepsy?"). For people with stereotyped recurrent severe seizures that can be easily recognized by the person's family, the drug diazepam is now available as a gel that can be administered rectally by a family member. This method of drug delivery may be able to stop prolonged seizures before they develop into status epilepticus.

For most people with epilepsy, seizures can be controlled with just one drug at the optimal dosage. Combining medications usually amplifies side effects such as fatigue and decreased appetite, so doctors usually prescribe *monotherapy*, or the use of just one drug, whenever possible. Combinations of drugs are sometimes prescribed if monotherapy fails to effectively control a patient's seizures.

The number of times a person needs to take medication each day is usually determined by the drug's half-life, or the time it takes for half the drug dose to be *metabolized* or broken down into other substances in the body. Some drugs, such as phenytoin and phenobarbital, only need to be taken once a day, while others such as valproate must be taken more frequently.

Most side effects of antiepileptic drugs are relatively minor, such as fatigue, dizziness, or weight gain. However, severe and life-threatening side effects such as allergic reactions can occur. Epilepsy medication also may predispose people to developing depression or psychoses. People with epilepsy should consult a doctor immediately if they develop any kind of rash while on medication, or if they find themselves depressed or otherwise unable to think in a rational manner. Other danger signs that should be discussed with a doctor immediately are extreme fatigue, staggering or other movement problems, and slurring of words. People with epilepsy should be aware that their epilepsy medication can interact with many other drugs in potentially harmful ways. For this reason, people with epilepsy should always tell doctors who treat them which medications they are taking. Women also should know that some antiepileptic drugs can interfere with the effectiveness of oral contraceptives, and they should discuss this possibility with their doctors.

Since people can become more sensitive to medications as they age, they should have their blood levels of medication checked occasionally to see if the dose needs to be adjusted. The effects of a particular medication also sometimes wear off over time, leading to an increase in seizures if the dose is not adjusted. People should know that some citrus fruit, in particular grapefruit juice, may interfere with breakdown of many drugs. This can cause too much of the drug to build up in their bodies, often worsening the side effects.

Tailoring the dosage of antiepileptic drugs

When a person starts a new epilepsy drug, it is important to tailor the dosage to achieve the best results. People's bodies react to medications in very different and sometimes unpredictable ways, so it may take some time to find the right drug at the right dose to provide optimal control of seizures while minimizing side effects. A drug that has no effect or very bad side effects at one dose may work very well at another dose. Doctors will usually prescribe a low dose of the new drug initially and monitor blood levels of the drug to determine when the best possible dose has been reached.

Generic versions are available for many antiepileptic drugs. The chemicals in generic drugs are exactly the same as in the brand-name drugs, but they may be absorbed or processed differently in the body because of the way they are prepared. Therefore, patients should always check with their doctors before switching to a generic version of their medication.

Discontinuing medication

Some doctors will advise people with epilepsy to discontinue their antiepileptic drugs after two years have passed without a seizure. Others feel it is better to wait for four to five years. Discontinuing medication should *only* be done with a doctor's advice and supervision. It is very important to continue taking epilepsy medication for as long as the doctor prescribes it. People also should ask the doctor or pharmacist ahead of time what they should do if they miss a dose. Discontinuing medication without a doctor's advice is one of the major reasons people who have been seizure-free begin having new seizures. Seizures that result from suddenly stopping medication can be very serious and can lead to status epilepticus. Furthermore, there is some evidence that uncontrolled seizures trigger changes in neurons that can make it more difficult to treat the seizures in the future.

The chance that a person will eventually be able to discontinue medication varies depending on the person's age and his or her type of epilepsy. More than half of children who go into remission with medication can eventually stop their medication without having new seizures. One study showed that 68 percent of adults who had been seizure-free for 2 years before stopping medication were able to do so without having more seizures and 75 percent could successfully discontinue medication if they had been seizure-free for 3 years. However, the odds of successfully stopping medication are not as good for people with a family history of epilepsy, those who need multiple medications, those with partial seizures, and those who continue to have abnormal EEG results while on medication.

SURGERY

When seizures cannot be adequately controlled by medications, doctors may recommend that the person be evaluated for surgery. Most surgery for epilepsy is performed by teams of doctors at medical centers. To decide if a person may benefit from surgery, doctors consider the type or types of seizures he or she has. They also take into account the brain region involved and how important that region is for everyday behavior. Surgeons usually avoid operating in areas of the brain that are necessary for speech, language, hearing, or other important abilities. Doctors may perform tests such as a WADA test (administration of the drug amobarbitol into the carotid artery) to find areas of the brain that control speech and memory. They often monitor the patient intensively prior to surgery in order to pinpoint the exact location in the brain where seizures begin. They also may use implanted electrodes to record brain activity from the surface of the brain. This yields better information than an external EEG.

A 1990 National Institutes of Health consensus conference on surgery for epilepsy concluded that there are three broad categories of epilepsy that can be treated successfully with surgery. These include partial seizures, seizures that begin as partial seizures before spreading to the rest of the brain, and unilateral multifocal epilepsy with infantile hemiplegia (such as Rasmussen's encephalitis). Doctors generally recommend surgery only after patients have tried two or three different medications without success, or if there is an identifiable brain *lesion*— a damaged or abnormally functioning area—believed to cause the seizures.

If a person is considered a good candidate for surgery and has seizures that cannot be controlled with available medication, experts generally agree that surgery should be performed as early as possible. It can be difficult for a person who has had years of seizures to fully re-adapt to a seizure-free life if the surgery is successful. The person may never have had an opportunity to develop independence and he or she may have had difficulties with school and work that could have been avoided with earlier treatment. Surgery should always be performed with support from rehabilitation specialists and counselors who can help the person deal with the many psychological, social, and employment issues he or she may face.

While surgery can significantly reduce or even halt seizures for some people, it is important to remember that any kind of surgery carries some amount of risk (usually small). Surgery for epilepsy does not always successfully reduce seizures and it can result in cognitive or personality changes, even in people who are excellent candidates for surgery. Patients should ask their surgeon about his or her experience, success rates, and complication rates with the procedure they are considering.

Even when surgery completely ends a person's seizures, it is important to continue taking seizure medication for some time to give the brain time to re-adapt. Doctors generally recommend medication for 2 years after a successful operation to avoid new seizures.

Surgery to treat underlying conditions

In cases where seizures are caused by a brain tumor, hydrocephalus, or other conditions that can be treated with surgery, doctors may operate to treat these underlying conditions. In many cases, once the underlying condition is success-fully treated, a person's seizures will stop as well.

Surgery to remove a seizure focus

The most common type of surgery for epilepsy is removal of a *seizure focus*, or small area of the brain where seizures originate. This type of surgery, which doctors may refer to as a *lobectomy* or *lesionectomy*, is appropriate only for partial seizures that originate in just one area of the brain. In general, people have a better chance of becoming seizure-free after surgery if they have a small, well-defined seizure focus. Lobectomies have a 55-70 percent success rate when the type of epilepsy and the seizure focus is well-defined. The most common type of lobectomy is a *temporal lobe resection,* which is performed for people with temporal lobe epilepsy. Temporal lobe resection leads to a significant reduction or complete cessation of seizures about 70 - 90 percent of the time.

Multiple subpial transection

When seizures originate in part of the brain that cannot be removed, surgeons may perform a procedure called a *multiple subpial transection*. In this type of operation, which was first described in 1989, surgeons make a series of cuts that are designed to prevent seizures from spreading into other parts of the brain while leaving the person's normal abilities intact. About 70 percent of patients who undergo a multiple subpial transection have satisfactory improvement in seizure control.

Corpus callosotomy

Corpus callosotomy, Corpus callosotomy, or severing the network of neural connections between the right and left halves, or *hemispheres,* of the brain, is done primarily in children with severe seizures that start in one half of the brain and spread to the other side. Corpus callosotomy can end drop attacks and other generalized seizures. However, the procedure does not stop seizures in the side of the brain where they originate, and these partial seizures may even increase after surgery.

Hemispherectomy

This procedure, which removes half of the brain's cortex, or outer layer, is used only for children who have Rasmussen's encephalitis or other severe damage to one brain hemisphere and who also have seizures that do not respond well to medication. While this type of surgery is very radical and is performed only as a last resort, children often recover very well from the procedure, and their seizures usually are greatly reduced or may cease altogether. With intense rehabilitation, they often recover nearly normal abilities. Since the chance of a full recovery is best in young children, hemispherectomy should be performed as early in a child's life as possible. It is almost never performed in children older than 13.

DEVICES

The vagus nerve stimulator was approved by the U.S. Food and Drug Administration (FDA) in 1997 for use in people with seizures that are not well-controlled by medication. The vagus nerve stimulator is a battery-powered device that is surgically implanted under the skin of the chest, much like a pacemaker, and is attached to the vagus nerve in the lower neck. This device delivers short bursts of electrical energy to the brain via the vagus nerve. On average, this stimulation reduces seizures by about 20-40 percent. Patients usually cannot stop taking epilepsy medication because of the stimulator, but they often experience fewer seizures and they may be able to reduce the dose of their medication. Side effects of the vagus nerve stimulator are generally mild, but may include ear pain, a sore throat, or nausea. Adjusting the amount of stimulation can usually eliminate these side effects. The batteries in the vagus nerve stimulator need to be replaced about once every 5 years; this requires a minor operation that can usually be performed as an outpatient procedure.

Several new devices may become available for epilepsy in the future. Researchers are studying whether *transcranial magnetic stimulation,* a procedure which uses a strong magnet held outside the head to influence brain activity, may reduce seizures. They also hope to develop implantable devices that can deliver drugs to specific parts of the brain.

Diet

Studies have shown that, in some cases, children may experience fewer seizures if they maintain a strict diet rich in fats and low in carbohydrates. This unusual diet, called the *ketogenic diet,* causes the body to break down fats instead of carbohydrates to survive. This condition is called ketosis. One study of 150 children whose seizures were poorly controlled by medication found that about one-fourth of the children had a 90 percent or better decrease in seizures with the ketogenic diet, and another half of the group had a 50 percent or better decrease in their seizures. Moreover, some children can discontinue the ketogenic diet after several years and remain seizure-free. The ketogenic diet is not easy to maintain, as it requires strict adherence to an unusual and limited range of foods. Possible side effects include retarded growth due to nutritional deficiency and a buildup of uric acid in the blood, which can lead to kidney stones. People who try the ketogenic diet should seek the guidance of a dietician to ensure that it does not lead to serious nutritional deficiency.

Researchers are not sure how ketosis inhibits seizures. One study showed that a byproduct of ketosis called beta-hydroxybutyrate (BHB) inhibits seizures in animals. If BHB also works in humans, researchers may eventually be able to develop drugs that mimic the seizure-inhibiting effects of the ketogenic diet.

Other Treatment Strategies

Researchers are studying whether biofeedback—a strategy in which individuals learn to control their own brain waves—may be useful in controlling seizures. However, this type of therapy is controversial and most studies have shown discouraging results. Taking large doses of vitamins generally does not help a person's seizures and may even be harmful in some cases. However, a good diet and some vitamin supplements, particularly folic acid, may help reduce some birth defects and medication-related nutritional deficiencies. Use of non-vitamin supplements such as melatonin is controversial and can be risky. One study showed that melatonin may reduce seizures in some children, while another found that the risk of seizures increased measurably with melatonin. Most non-vitamin supplements such as those found in health food stores are not regulated by the FDA, so their true effects and their interactions with other drugs are largely unknown.

3.10 How Does Epilepsy Affect Daily Life?

Most people with epilepsy lead outwardly normal lives. Approximately 80 percent can be significantly helped by modern therapies, and some may go months or years between seizures. However, epilepsy can and does affect daily life for people with epilepsy, their families, and their friends. People with severe seizures that resist treatment have, on average, a shorter life expectancy and an increased risk of cognitive impairment, particularly if the seizures developed in early childhood. These impairments may be related to the underlying conditions that cause epilepsy or to epilepsy treatment rather than the epilepsy itself.

Behavior and Emotions

It is not uncommon for people with epilepsy, especially children, to develop behavioral and emotional problems. Sometimes these problems are caused by embarrassment or frustration associated with epilepsy. Other problems may result from bullying, teasing, or avoidance in school and other social settings. In children, these problems can be minimized if parents encourage a positive outlook and independence, do not reward negative behavior with unusual amounts of attention, and try to stay attuned to their child's needs and feelings. Families must learn to accept and live with the seizures without blaming or resenting the affected person. Counseling services can help families cope with epilepsy in a positive manner. Epilepsy support groups also can help by providing a way for people with epilepsy and their family members to share their experiences, frustrations, and tips for coping with the disorder.

People with epilepsy have an increased risk of poor self-esteem, depression, and suicide. These problems may be a reaction to a lack of understanding or discomfort about epilepsy that may result in cruelty or avoidance by other people. Many people with epilepsy also live with an ever-present fear that they will have another seizure.

Driving and Recreation

For many people with epilepsy, the risk of seizures restricts their independence, in particular the ability to drive. Most states and the District of Columbia will not issue a driver's license to someone with epilepsy unless the person can document that they have gone a specific amount of time without a seizure (the waiting period varies from a few months to several years). Some states make exceptions for this policy when seizures don't impair consciousness, occur only during sleep, or have long auras or other warning signs that allow the person to avoid driving when a seizure is likely to occur. Studies show that the risk of having a seizure-related accident decreases as the length of time since the last seizure increases. One study found that the risk of having a seizure-related motor vehicle accident is 93 percent less in people who wait at least 1 year after their last seizure before driving, compared to people who wait for shorter intervals.

The risk of seizures also restricts people's recreational choices. For instance, people with epilepsy should not participate in sports such as skydiving or motor racing where a moment's inattention could lead to injury. Other activities, such as swimming and sailing, should be done only with precautions and/or supervision. However, jogging, football, and many other sports are reasonably safe for a person with epilepsy. Studies to date have not shown any increase in seizures due to sports, although these studies have not focused on any activity in particular. There is some evidence that regular exercise may even improve seizure control in some people. Sports are often such a positive factor in life that it is best for the person to participate, although the person with epilepsy and the coach or other leader should take appropriate safety precautions. It is important to take steps to avoid potential sports-related problems such as dehydration, overexertion, and hypoglycemia, as these problems can increase the risk of seizures.

EDUCATION AND EMPLOYMENT

By law, people with epilepsy or other handicaps in the United States cannot be denied employment or access to any educational, recreational, or other activity because of their seizures. However, one survey showed that only about 56 percent of people with epilepsy finish high school and about 15 percent finish college—rates much lower than those for the general population. The same survey found that about 25 percent of working-age people with epilepsy are unemployed. These numbers indicate that significant barriers still exist for people with epilepsy in school and work. Restrictions on driving limit the employment opportunities for many people with epilepsy, and many find it difficult to face the misunderstandings and social pressures they encounter in public situations. Antiepileptic drugs also may cause side effects that interfere with concentration and memory. Children with epilepsy may need extra time to complete schoolwork, and they sometimes may need to have instructions or other information repeated for them. Teachers should be told what to do if a child in their classroom has a seizure, and parents should work with the school system to find reasonable ways to accommodate any special needs their child may have.

PREGNANCY AND MOTHERHOOD

Women with epilepsy are often concerned about whether they can become pregnant and have a healthy child. This is usually possible. While some seizure medications and some types of epilepsy may reduce a person's interest in sexual activity, most people with epilepsy can become pregnant. Moreover, women with epilepsy have a 90 percent or better chance of having a normal, healthy baby, and the risk of birth defects is only about 4-6 percent. The risk that children of parents with epilepsy will develop epilepsy themselves is only about 5 percent unless the parent has a clearly hereditary form of the disorder. Parents who are worried that their epilepsy may be hereditary may wish to consult a genetic counselor to determine what the risk might be. Amniocentesis and high-level ultrasound can be performed during pregnancy to ensure that the baby is developing normally, and a procedure called a maternal serum alpha-fetoprotein test can be used for prenatal diagnosis of many conditions if a problem is suspected.

There are several precautions women can take before and during pregnancy to reduce the risks associated with pregnancy and delivery. Women who are thinking about becoming pregnant should talk with their doctors to learn any special risks associated with their epilepsy and the medications they may be taking. Some seizure medications, particularly valproate, trimethadione, and phenytoin, are known to increase the risk of having a child with birth defects such as cleft palate, heart problems, or finger and toe defects. For this reason, a woman's doctor may advise switching to other medications during pregnancy. Whenever possible, a woman should allow her doctor enough time to properly change medications, including phasing in the new medications and checking to determine when blood levels are stabilized, before she tries to become pregnant. Women should also begin prenatal vitamin supplements—especially with folic acid, which may reduce the risk of some birth defects—well before pregnancy. Women who discover that they are pregnant but have not already spoken with their doctor about ways to reduce the risks should do so as soon as possible. However, they should continue taking seizure medication as prescribed until that time to avoid preventable seizures. Seizures during pregnancy can harm the developing baby or lead to miscarriage, particularly if the seizures are severe. Nevertheless, many women who have seizures during pregnancy have normal, healthy babies.

Women with epilepsy sometimes experience a change in their seizure frequency during pregnancy, even if they do not change medications. About 25 to 40 percent of women have an increase in their seizure frequency while they are pregnant, while other women may have fewer seizures during pregnancy. The frequency of seizures during pregnancy may be influenced by a variety of factors, including the woman's increased blood volume during pregnancy, which can dilute the effect of medication. Women should have their blood levels of seizure medications monitored closely during and after pregnancy, and the medication dosage should be adjusted accordingly.

Pregnant women with epilepsy should take prenatal vitamins and get plenty of sleep to avoid seizures caused by sleep deprivation. They also should take vitamin K supplements after 34 weeks of pregnancy to reduce the risk of a blood-clotting disorder in infants called neonatal coagulopathy that can result from fetal exposure to epilepsy medications. Finally, they should get good prenatal care, avoid tobacco, caffeine, alcohol, and illegal drugs, and try to avoid stress.

Labor and delivery usually proceed normally for women with epilepsy, although there is a slightly increased risk of hemorrhage, eclampsia, premature labor, and cesarean section. Doctors can administer antiepileptic drugs intravenously and monitor blood levels of anticonvulsant medication during labor to reduce the risk that the labor will trigger a seizure. Babies sometimes have symptoms of withdrawal from the mother's seizure medication after they are born, but these problems wear off in a few weeks or months and usually do not cause serious or long-term effects. A mother's blood levels of anticonvulsant medication should be checked frequently after delivery as medication often needs to be decreased.

Epilepsy medications need not influence a woman's decision about breast-feeding her baby. Only minor amounts of epilepsy medications are secreted in breast milk; usually not enough to harm the baby and much less than the baby was exposed to in the womb. On rare occasions, the baby may become excessively drowsy or feed poorly, and these problems should be closely monitored. However, experts believe the benefits of breast-feeding outweigh the risks except in rare circumstances.

To increase doctors' understanding of how different epilepsy medications affect pregnancy and the chances of having a healthy baby, Massachusetts General Hospital has begun a nationwide registry for women who take antiepileptic drugs while pregnant. Women who enroll in this program are given educational materials on pre-conception planning and perinatal care and are asked to provide information about the health of their children (this information is kept confidential). Women and physicians can contact this registry by calling 1-888-233-2334 or 617-726-7739 (fax: 617-724-8307).

Women with epilepsy should be aware that some epilepsy medications can interfere with the effectiveness of oral contraceptives. Women who wish to use oral contraceptives to prevent pregnancy should discuss this with their doctors, who may be able to prescribe a different kind of antiepileptic medication or suggest other ways of avoiding an unplanned pregnancy.

3.11 ARE THERE SPECIAL RISKS ASSOCIATED WITH EPILEPSY?

Although most people with epilepsy lead full, active lives, they are at special risk for two life-threatening conditions: status epilepticus and sudden unexplained death.

STATUS EPILEPTICUS

Status epilepticus is a severe, life-threatening condition in which a person either has prolonged seizures or does not fully regain consciousness between seizures. The amount of time in a prolonged seizure that must pass before a person should be diagnosed with status epilepticus is a subject of debate. Many doctors now diagnose status epilepticus if a person has been in a prolonged seizure for 5 minutes. However, other doctors use more conservative definitions of this condition and may not diagnose status epilepticus unless the person has had a prolonged seizure of 10 minutes or even 30 minutes.

Status epilepticus affects about 195,000 people each year in the United States and results in about 42,000 deaths. While people with epilepsy are at an increased risk for status epilepticus, about 60 percent of people who develop this condition have no previous seizure history. These cases often result from tumors, trauma, or other problems that affect the brain and may themselves be life-threatening.

While most seizures do not require emergency medical treatment, someone with a prolonged seizure lasting more than 5 minutes may be in status epilepticus and should be taken to an emergency room immediately. It is important to treat a person with status epilepticus as soon as possible. One study showed that 80 percent of people in status epilepticus who received medication within 30 minutes of seizure onset eventually stopped having seizures, whereas only 40 percent recovered if 2 hours had passed before they received medication. Doctors in a hospital setting can treat status epilepticus with several different drugs and can undertake emergency life-saving measures, such as administering oxygen, if necessary.

People in status epilepticus do not always have severe convulsive seizures. Instead, they may have repeated or prolonged nonconvulsive seizures. This type of status epilepticus may appear as a sustained episode of confusion or agitation in someone who does not ordinarily have that kind of mental impairment. While this type of episode may not seem as severe as convulsive status epilepticus, it should still be treated as an emergency.

SUDDEN UNEXPLAINED DEATH

For reasons that are poorly understood, people with epilepsy have an increased risk of dying suddenly for no discernible reason. This condition, called *sudden unexplained death*, can occur in people without epilepsy, but epilepsy increases the risk about two-fold. Researchers are still unsure why sudden unexplained death occurs. One study suggested that use of more than two anticonvulsant drugs may be a risk factor. However, it is not clear whether the use of multiple drugs causes the sudden death, or whether people who use multiple anticonvulsants have a greater risk of death because they have more severe types of epilepsy.

3.12 WHAT RESEARCH IS BEING DONE ON EPILEPSY?

While research has led to many advances in understanding and treating epilepsy, there are many unanswered questions about how and why seizures develop, how they can best be treated or prevented, and how they influence other brain activity and brain development. Researchers, many of whom are supported by the

National Institute of Neurological Disorders and Stroke (NINDS), are studying all of these questions. They also are working to identify and test new drugs and other treatments for epilepsy and to learn how those treatments affect brain activity and development. NINDS' Epilepsy Therapeutics Research Program studies potential antiepileptic drugs with the goal of enhancing treatment for epilepsy. Since it began in 1975, this program has screened more than 22,000 compounds for their potential as antiepileptic drugs and has contributed to the development of five drugs that are now approved for use in the United States as well as others that are still being developed or tested.

Scientists continue to study how excitatory and inhibitory neurotransmitters interact with brain cells to control nerve firing. They can apply different chemicals to cultures of neurons in laboratory dishes to study how those chemicals influence neuronal activity. They also are studying how glia and other non-neuronal cells in the brain contribute to seizures. This research may lead to new drugs and other new ways of treating seizures.

Researchers also are working to identify genes that may influence epilepsy in some way. Identifying these genes can reveal the underlying chemical processes that influence epilepsy and point to new ways of preventing or treating this disorder. Researchers also can study rats and mice that have missing or abnormal copies of certain genes to determine how these genes affect normal brain development and resistance to damage from disease and other environmental factors. Researchers may soon be able to use devices called gene chips to determine each person's genetic makeup or to learn which genes are active. This information may allow doctors to prevent epilepsy or to predict which treatments will be most beneficial.

Doctors are now experimenting with several new types of therapies for epilepsy. In one preliminary clinical trial, doctors have begun transplanting fetal pig neurons that produce GABA into the brains of patients to learn whether the cell transplants can help control seizures. Preliminary research suggests that stem cell transplants also may prove beneficial for treating epilepsy. Research showing that the brain undergoes subtle changes prior to a seizure has led to a prototype device that may be able to predict seizures up to 3 minutes before they begin. If this device works, it could greatly reduce the risk of injury from seizures by allowing people to move to a safe area before their seizures start. This type of device also may be hooked up to a treatment pump or other device that will automatically deliver an antiepileptic drug or an electric impulse to forestall the seizures.

Researchers are continually improving MRI and other brain scans. Pre-surgical brain imaging can guide doctors to abnormal brain tissue and away from essential parts of the brain. Researchers also are using brain scans such as magnetoencephalograms (MEG) and magnetic resonance spectroscopy (MRS) to identify and study subtle problems in the brain that cannot otherwise be detected. Their findings may lead to a better understanding of epilepsy and how it can be treated.

3.13 What To Do If You See Someone Having a Seizure

If you see someone having a seizure with convulsions and/or loss of consciousness, here's how you can help:

1.   Roll the person on his or her side to prevent choking on any fluids or vomit.
2.   Cushion the person's head.
3.   Loosen any tight clothing around the neck.
4.   Keep the person's airway open. If necessary, grip the person's jaw gently and tilt his or her head back.
5.   Do NOT restrict the person from moving unless he or she is in danger.
6.   Do NOT put anything into the person's mouth, not even medicine or liquid. These can cause choking or damage to the person's jaw, tongue, or teeth. Contrary to widespread belief, people cannot swallow their tongues during a seizure or any other time.
7.   Remove any sharp or solid objects that the person might hit during the seizure.
8.   Note how long the seizure lasts and what symptoms occurred so you can tell a doctor or emergency personnel if necessary.
9.   Stay with the person until the seizure ends.

Call 911 if:

- The person is pregnant or has diabetes.
- The seizure happened in water.
- The seizure lasts longer than 5 minutes.
- The person does not begin breathing again and return to consciousness after the seizure stops.
- Another seizure starts before the person regains consciousness.
- The person injures himself or herself during the seizure.
- This is a first seizure or you think it might be. If in doubt, check to see if the person has a medical identification card or jewelry stating that he or she has epilepsy or a seizure disorder.

After the seizure ends, the person will probably be groggy and tired. He or she also may have a headache and be confused or embarrassed. Be patient with the person and try to help him or her find a place to rest if he or she is tired or doesn't feel well. If necessary, offer to call a taxi, a friend, or a relative to help the person get home safely.

If you see someone having a non-convulsive seizure, remember that the person's behavior is not intentional. The person may wander aimlessly or make alarming or unusual gestures. You can help by following these guidelines:

1. Remove any dangerous objects from the area around the person or in his or her path.
2. Don't try to stop the person from wandering unless he or she is in danger.
3. Don't shake the person or shout.
4. Stay with the person until he or she is completely alert.

3.14 CONCLUSION

Many people with epilepsy lead productive and outwardly normal lives. Many medical and research advances in the past two decades have led to a better understanding of epilepsy and seizures than ever before. Advanced brain scans and other techniques allow greater accuracy in diagnosing epilepsy and determining when a patient may be helped by surgery. More than 20 different medications and a variety of surgical techniques are now available and provide good control of seizures for most people with epilepsy. Other treatment options include the ketogenic diet and the first implantable device, the vagus nerve stimulator. Research on the underlying causes of epilepsy, including identification of genes for some forms of epilepsy and febrile seizures, has led to a greatly improved understanding of epilepsy that may lead to more effective treatments

4

GENERAL REFERENCE

4.1 GENERAL SITES

4E-0004
Epilepsy Foundation: Online Center for Clinical Care
Visitors to this Web page will find a broad array of epilepsy resources. Fact sheets are provided in sections on assessment, treatment, planning, special populations, and professional resources. The "Assessment" section offers information on seizure types, epileptic syndromes, impact on the individual and family, education and vocation, and recommendations for referral. In the "Treatment" section there is information on antiepileptic drugs, surgery, diet, and alternative therapies. Tips on vocation, education, self-management, and stress reduction are featured in the "Planning Section." Information for older patients, women, alcoholics, and people with developmental disabilities is found in the Populations section. In addition, information is provided on the Gene Discovery Project, and there are related links in the "Resources" section.
http://www.efa.org/clinicalcare/index.html

4E-0001
Epilepsy.com Epilepsy.com offers a broad array of resources related to epilepsy. The site is best navigated through a drop-down menu that allows visitors to go directly to a health library and a "From Our Experts" section. The library is comprehensive and offers detailed fact sheets on epilepsy, medications, surgery, lifestyle, safety, and employment. There are also fact sheets for special populations, such as children, women, and seniors. Related resources are provided. In the "Expert" section, there are answers to common concerns such as flashing lights and seizures, pregnancy, and driving. Pharmacists also answer common questions about medications.
http://www.epilepsy.com

4E-0076
EpilepsyLife.com This comprehensive Web page for people living with epilepsy offers e-mail support groups, chat rooms, articles on epilepsy, and the latest epilepsy news. Book recommendations, personal stories, and links to related resources are also featured. http://www.epilepsylife.com

`4E-0002`   **MEDLINEplus: Epilepsy**   Resources on epilepsy are featured on this site, maintained by the National Library of Medicine. The site includes overviews of epilepsy, news, alternative therapies, clinical trials, diagnostic tests, and disease management. There is also information on nutrition, research, treatment, and specific conditions such as pregnancy and epilepsy. Special sections are dedicated to children, seniors, teenagers, and women.
http://www.nlm.nih.gov/medlineplus/epilepsy.html

`4E-0003`   **New York Online Access to Health (NOAH): Epilepsy**   A comprehensive listing of Internet resources related to epilepsy is featured on this Web page, maintained by NOAH (New York Online Access to Health). Seventy-five sites are listed in categories such as "What is Epilepsy," care and treatment, complications and related concerns, research, and information resources.
http://www.noah-health.org/english/illness/neuro/epilepsy.html

4.2 News and Headlines

`4E-0005`   **Epilepsy Foundation: EpilepsyUSA Magazine**   Recent full-text articles from the Epilepsy Foundation's *EpilepsyUSA* magazine are featured on this site. In addition, articles from previous issues are available in their online archive. There is also a link for the biannual publication, *Between Us,* for women with epilepsy.
http://www.efa.org/epusa/index.html

`4E-0006`   **Medscape: Epilepsy**   Articles, conference summaries, treatment updates, and practice guidelines related to epilepsy are featured on this Web site. A free registration is required to access the articles. (free registration)
http://www.medscape.com/server-java/SearchClinical?QueryText=epilepsy

`4E-0007`   **Reuters Health**   The latest health news is offered on this Web site, courtesy of Reuters Ltd. For information specific to epilepsy, visitors must click on the "Search" icon and enter "epilepsy." The results will show the most recent stories, with a notation for professional medical news, industry briefing, and health eLine (news for the consumer). The search can also be limited to consumer news. While browsing the medical news headlines is free, there is a small fee to view a full-text professional medical news article or a health eLine story that is more than 30 days old.
(some features fee-based) http://www.reutershealth.com

4.3 Journals

4E-0008 | **Epilepsia** Information on the International League Against Epilepsy's journal, *Epilepsia,* is featured on this Web page. The purpose of the journal, instructions for authors, reprint availability, and subscription information are provided. In addition, a free sample copy is available upon request.
(fee-based) http://www.blackwellscience.com/journals/epilepsia/

4E-0077 | **Epilepsy Abstracts** Abstracts of epilepsy journal articles, drawn from more than 4,000 leading international biomedical journals, are featured in this journal. An online sample copy can be viewed in Adobe Acrobat reader. (fee-based)
http://www.elsevier.com/locate/inca/506013

4E-0009 | **Epilepsy and Behavior** A journal titled *Epilepsy & Behavior* is featured on this Web page. Visitors can access full-text articles in the current issue by choosing "Current Issue" from the "Content" drop-down menu. Articles from back issues are available for purchase, or free for subscribers. A short list of related Web sites is provided. (some features fee-based) http://www.apnet.com/eb

4E-0010 | **Epilepsy Research** Information on the journal *Epilepsy Research* is provided on this site, hosted by the publisher Elsevier Science. A free sample copy can be viewed on the site. Subscription information is provided. (some features fee-based)
http://www.elsevier.nl/inca/publications/store/5/0/6/0/5/3/

4E-0011 | **National Epifellows Foundation: Epilepsy Quarterly** The quarterly newsletter of the National Epifellows Foundation is provided on this Web site. The entire newsletter is available for download in PDF format. Newsletters date back to 1993.
http://www.epifellows.com/EQRT/EQTOC.html

4E-0012 | **Seizure** Visitors to this site will find academic articles focused on epilepsy from the international journal *Seizure.* Abstracts are available online for the current issue as well as archives dating back to 1996. Full-text articles are available at no charge to subscribers or for a fee to others.
(some features fee-based)
http://www.harcourt-international.com/journals/seiz/

4.4 Article and Abstract Searches Online

4E-0013 | **Docguide.com** News, Webcasts, and case studies for a variety of health topics are provided on this Web site. The information is

directed to healthcare professionals but may be of interest to consumers seeking technical information. Visitors can access items specific to epilepsy by choosing "Epilepsy" from the "Select a Channel" drop-down menu at the top of the site. Reviews of articles recently published in medical journals are featured; access to the full-text of the original article requires a fee.
(some features fee-based) http://www.docguide.com

| 4E-0014 | **National Library of Medicine: PubMed** For those interested in highly technical journal research on epilepsy, PubMed offers an efficient search tool for citations of professional articles. Developed by the National Library of Medicine, the PubMed database contains more than 11 million citations, most with abstracts. Some citations also include links to full-text articles and related resources. http://www4.ncbi.nlm.nih.gov/PubMed/

4.5 ONLINE COMMUNITIES, FORUMS, AND LISTSERVS

| 4E-0015 | **Epilepsy Circle of Support** Developed by Ted Bergeron, the Epilepsy Circle of Support Web site offers many resources for epilepsy support. There are sections of the site dedicated to parents of children with epilepsy, children with epilepsy, and friends of people with epilepsy. Each section has a chat room, discussion boards, a newsletter, and articles. Other resources include an epilepsy e-mail list, a recognition page for those who have helped children with epilepsy, information on seizure service dogs, a bill of rights for children with epilepsy, a medicine database, and recommended books. In addition, there are related links.
http://members.tripod.com/~Ted_Bergeron/epilepsyhome.html

| 4E-0016 | **Epilepsy Foundation: eCommunity** An "eCommunity" (electronic community) has been created on this Web site by the Epilepsy Foundation. After a free registration process, visitors can access chat rooms, view discussion boards, and attend online chat events with experts. There are four interest groups: women and epilepsy, parents helping parents, teens, and living well with seizures. (free registration) http://206.239.147.40/ecommunities/

| 4E-0017 | **Epilepsy Support Group** Described as an e-mail-based support group, this site offers access to an epilepsy LISTSERV. The LISTSERV is open to people with epilepsy, parents of children with epilepsy, family and friends, and health professionals.
http://home.ease.lsoft.com/Archives/Epilepsy-L.html

| 4E-0018 | **Massachusetts General Hospital: Epilepsy Discussion Board** A message board dedicated to epilepsy is featured on this

Web site. The most recent topics are listed on this page topics from previous days can be accessed through a drop-down menu. A free registration process is required to post to the board.

(free registration)

http://neuro-mancer.mgh.harvard.edu/cgi-bin/forumdisplay.cgi?
action=topics&forum=Epilepsy&number=33&DaysPrune=20&LastLogin=

4.6 ASSOCIATIONS AND FOUNDATIONS

4E-0019   **American Academy of Neurology**   Although the academy's Web site is primarily directed to healthcare professionals, consumers may still find items related to epilepsy of interest. Under the "Patient Information" section, the full-text of the newsletter, *Neurovista,* is available, as well as a patient brochure entitled *What Is Epilepsy?* By choosing "Epilepsy" in the drop-down menu of the "Patient Info Guide," support groups, news stories, and a directory of neurologists are found. For more technical information, the "Clinical and Practice Info" section offers practice guidelines, including the full text of the "AAN Practice Guidelines." A variety of guidelines are available in this section including a practice advisory for the use of felbamate in epilepsy and practice parameters for antiepileptic drugs in brain tumors, discontinuing medications for seizure-free patients, and management issues for women with epilepsy.

http://www.aan.com/

4E-0020   **American Epilepsy Society**   This site is primarily directed to healthcare professionals, but consumers may still find useful information on epilepsy news, research, and related Internet links. The site contains information on research awards, research collaboration, online educational materials (some with CME credit), and publications. A link to NeuroCentral offers professionals information on current research activities and abstracts. The "Patient Care" section offers drug information and news. In addition, there is information on practice management.

http://www.aesnet.org

4E-0021   **Epilepsy Education Association, Inc.**   Dedicated to educating the public about epilepsy, the Epilepsy Education Association site offers online publications for general information about epilepsy, drug therapy, lifestyle changes, epilepsy and pregnancy, and surgical treatment. The publications contain illustrations that complement the text. In addition, there is a comprehensive list of related Internet resources for general information, clinical trials, and major medical centers with epilepsy programs.

http://www.iupui.edu/~epilepsy/

| 4E-0022 | **Epilepsy Foundation** A wealth of resources for patients, and their families, coping with epilepsy is featured on this site. Under the "AnswerPlace" section, there is detailed information on treatment, medications, surgery, and the ketogenic diet. Other topics covered include first aid, driving, employment, and insurance. The site also contains research information, including grant opportunities, clinical trials, and a pregnancy registry. The foundation's services are described, such as their public education programs, advocacy, support groups, and employment assistance. A link for local affiliates offers a directory of more than 40 chapters throughout the United States. Full-text articles and archives from their magazine, *EpilepsyUSA,* are also found on this site. In addition, the "eCommunities" section offers chat rooms and discussion groups. A "Marketplace" section allows visitors to make online purchases of books, manuals, brochures, and videos related to epilepsy.
http://www.efa.org

| 4E-0023 | **Epilepsy Institute** The Epilepsy Institute is dedicated to improving the quality of life for people with epilepsy. Their Web page offers a comprehensive fact sheet on epilepsy (also in Spanish) that covers causes, symptoms, diagnosis, treatment, first aid for seizures, and seizure prevention. There are also FAQs, information on studies on seizure alert dogs, and a comprehensive listing of links. Under the "News and Information" section, there is information on clinical trials, epilepsy events in New York City, and epilepsy news. Services such as counseling, education, employment, and stress management are offered for residents of New York City and Westchester County.
http://www.epilepsyinstitute.org

| 4E-0024 | **National Epifellows Foundation** The National Epifellows Foundation site offers information on professional conferences and research grants for the study of epilepsy. Consumers may find the *Epilepsy Quarterly* newsletter on the site of interest (PDF format). http://www.epifellows.com/

MEDICAL ASPECTS

5.1 CAUSES AND RISK FACTORS

4E-0026 **New York University, Mount Sinai Comprehensive Epilepsy Center: Causes and Risk Factors** An overview of epilepsy is provided on this site, which includes information such as the number of people with epilepsy and the age at which they get it. Causes of epilepsy are described, along with risk factors. There is also a discussion of hereditary influences and epilepsy. The prognosis for patients with epilepsy, including the risk of recurrent seizures after a first seizure, is explained, as well as remission of epilepsy and the risk of relapse. The effect of epilepsy on life span is addressed, as well as fatal seizures and unexplained death. http://epilepsy.med.nyu.edu/Book/cause.html

4E-0027 **PersonalMD.com: Epilepsy** A guide to epilepsy is featured on this Web page, courtesy of PersonalMD.com. The guide offers an explanation of what a seizure is and what is happening in the body during a seizure. Generalized and partial seizures are described. Epilepsy is also described, along with its causes and diagnostic tests, such as the electroencephalogram.
http://www.personalmd.com/healthtopics/crs/epilepsy.shtml

4E-0028 **University of Iowa: Causes of Epilepsy** The causes of epilepsy in young children are described on this Web page. Visitors can navigate through the causes by clicking on the icons at the top of the page. Causes include fever, brain injury before or during birth, brain injury after birth, and congenital malformations.
http://www.medicine.uiowa.edu/uhs/epilepsy/causes/cause1.html

5.2 DIAGNOSTIC PROCEDURES

4E-0029 **Epilepsy.com: Diagnosis of Epilepsy** By clicking on "Making the Diagnosis of Epilepsy," visitors can access an article on epilepsy diagnosis. Diagnostic tests are described, such as the electroencephalogram, blood tests, and the electrocardiogram, along with imaging tests, such as computed tomography and positron emission tomography. Other conditions that resemble epilepsy are discussed including sleep apnea, hypoglycemia, and panic attacks. http://www.epilepsy.com/gen_info.html

5.3 SEIZURE EDUCATION

4E-0030   **Epilepsy Foundation: Partial Seizures**   A collection of fact sheets related to partial seizures is provided on this site. Seizure types are described, along with simple partial seizures and complex partial seizures. Additional information on the site includes fact sheets on what complex partial seizures look like, dealing with other people, things to remember, handling partial seizures, and what causes partial seizures. There is also information on treating partial seizures and living with partial seizures.
http://www.efa.org/answerplace/getsection.cfm?keyname=partial

4E-0031   **Epilepsy Foundation: Seizures**   A variety of resources related to seizures are provided on this Web page. There is a seizure recognition chart that describes a seizure, what to do, and what not to do for seizures such as generalized tonic-clonic, absence, simple partial, complex partial, atonic, myoclonic, and infantile spasms. Additional fact sheets are provided for detailed descriptions of seizure types, knowing the symptoms of a seizure, and dealing with other people. There are also fact sheets on seizure recognition specifically for babysitters and teachers.
http://www.efa.org/answerplace/getsection.cfm?keyname=recognition

4E-0032   **University of Iowa: Types of Seizures**   Part of the Epilepsy in Young Children Web page, this site offers information on a variety of seizures, including generalized seizures, such as absence, myoclonic, atonic/tonic, and generalized tonic-clonic seizures, and partial seizures, such as simple partial and complex partial seizures. By clicking on the type of seizure, additional information, such as symptoms, and the prognosis for the child, is provided.
http://www.medicine.uiowa.edu/uhs/epilepsy/types/type.html

5.4 SYNDROMES AND CLASSIFICATIONS

4E-0033   **American Academy of Pediatrics: Febrile Seizures**   Information on febrile seizures—seizures that affect children between six months and five years old—is featured on this site. A definition of a febrile seizure is provided, along with what to do during a febrile seizure, the risk of having more seizures, and the chances of developing epilepsy. Treatment for febrile seizures is also described.
http://www.medem.com/search/article_display.cfm?
path=n:&mstr=/ZZZ4PU1JUSC.html&soc=AAP&srch_typ=NAV_SERCH

4E-0034 | **Epilepsy Syndromes** Developed by neurologist Dr. Michael Wei-Liang Chee, this Web site offers a guide to epilepsy syndromes. Presented in outline form, brief descriptions are provided for syndromes, such as benign myoclonic epilepsy in infants, juvenile myoclonic epilepsy, childhood absence epilepsy, juvenile absence epilepsy, and epilepsy with generalized tonic-clonic seizures in childhood. Additional syndromes covered include West's syndrome, Lennox-Gastaut syndrome, and progressive myoclonus epilepsies.
http://home.earthlink.net/~mchee1/episynd.html

4E-0036 | **National Institute of Neurological Disorders and Stroke (NINDS): Febrile Seizures** Febrile seizures, convulsions caused by a fever in infants or young children, are described on this site. The site offers parents tips on what to do during a seizure and explains treatment, prognosis, and ongoing research of the condition. In addition, there are links on the left side of the page for more information on febrile seizures such as ongoing clinical trials, research literature, and news.
http://www.ninds.nih.gov/
health_and_medical/disorders/febrile_seizures.htm

4E-0037 | **National Institute of Neurological Disorders and Stroke (NINDS): Infantile Spasms** Visitors to this site will find a fact sheet on infantile spasms (IS). IS is described, along with its treatment and prognosis for the infant. A bibliography, and resources for related information are provided. In addition, there is a link for clinical trial information, and for researching the medical literature on this topic.
http://www.ninds.nih.gov/
health_and_medical/disorders/infantilespasms.htm

4E-0038 | **Tuberous Sclerosis Association: Epilepsy in Tuberous Sclerosis** The Tuberous Sclerosis Association offers this publication on epilepsy in tuberous sclerosis. The fact sheet explains that epilepsy is one of the most common features of tuberous sclerosis. A detailed description of epilepsy is provided, along with information on several types of seizures. In addition, an explanation is provided of why epilepsy occurs in tuberous sclerosis.
http://www.tuberous-sclerosis.org/publications/epilepsy.htm

5.5 THERAPIES AND TREATMENTS

GENERAL RESOURCES

4E-0039 **Epilepsy Foundation: Treatment Options** This comprehensive site offers a variety of fact sheets on treatment options. Visitors will find more than 30 fact sheets covering topics such as medicines for epilepsy, partial seizures, surgery, nontraditional therapies, and vagus nerve stimulation. A section entitled "You and Your Treatment" takes patients through an in-depth tutorial covering medical history, diagnostic tests, and the various treatment options. Tips on talking to one's doctor and managing seizures are also provided.
http://www.efa.org/answerplace/getsection.cfm?keyname=treatment

4E-0040 **University of Iowa: Epilepsy Therapies** Drawn from an Epilepsy in Young Children Web page, this site focuses on treatment options. The site can be navigated by clicking on the treatment option on the top of the page; options include anticonvulsant medications, ketogenic diet, surgery, and vagal nerve stimulator. In the "Medications" section, there is a list of drugs provided with hyperlinks for additional information on the drug and its side effects. A link found in the vagal nerve stimulator section offers detailed information on the technique from the New York Hospital-Cornell Medical Center.
http://www.medicine.uiowa.edu/uhs/epilepsy/therapy/treat.html

DRUG THERAPIES

4E-0041 **Epilepsy Foundation: Treatment with Medications** A fact sheet is featured on this site covering commonly prescribed medications to prevent seizures, as well as newer drugs. Side effects of medication and the possibility of needing more than one drug are examined. Links are also available for further information on tests during treatment, treatment during pregnancy, and non-drug treatment options.
http://www.efa.org/answerplace/treatment/treatment.html

4E-0042 **New York University, Mount Sinai Comprehensive Epilepsy Center: Antiepileptic Drug Therapy** Detailed information on antiepileptic drug therapy is featured on this Web page. The site describes the time required for medications to work, the goals of drug therapy, and when to start treatment. Factors to consider when choosing a primary treatment drug and secondary drugs are addressed. Side effects, and the need to monitor blood levels, are also discussed. In addition, the interaction between antiepileptic drugs and birth control pills, alcohol, and other drugs is described. Generic versus brand name drugs are discussed, as well as newly approved drugs. Drugs currently under investigation are also described.

http://epilepsy.med.nyu.edu/Book/aedtx.html

KETOGENIC DIET

4E-0043 | **Epilepsy Foundation: Ketogenic Diet** An article on the use of the ketogenic diet as therapy for children with epilepsy is provided on this Web page. The process of placing a child on the diet, as well as that of maintaining the diet, is described. Current research findings on the diet are outlined, such as the fact that the diet produces success rates similar to medication and that it appears effective for every seizure type. Further research needs for a "keto" pill are examined. Side effects and difficulties associated with the diet are also described.

http://www.efa.org/answerplace/epusa/ketogenic.html

4E-0044 | **Johns Hopkins Medicine: Ketogenic Diet Fact Sheet** A fact sheet on the ketogenic diet for children with epilepsy is provided on this site. The diet is described, along with information on who can be helped by the diet and how effective the diet may be for a patient. Common concerns are addressed such as the quality of the diet for children, the risk of high-fat diets and heart disease, and complications. A video and book on the ketogenic diet are available for purchase from the site. In addition, news items related to the ketogenic diet are provided.

http://www.hopkinsmedicine.org/ketodiet.html

SEIZURE SURGERY

4E-0045 | **Epilepsy Foundation: Surgery Therapy** Information on surgery for the control of seizures is provided on this Web page. Several types of surgery are described, including lobectomy, hemispherectomy, corpus callosotomy, and multiple subpial transection. A description of each type of operation along with presurgical testing is presented, benefits and risks, costs, and planning for surgery. Vagus nerve stimulation—is also examined in detail, with information on the operation, monitoring treatment, handling the magnet, costs, and efficacy.

http://www.efa.org/answerplace/getsection.cfm?keyname=surgery

4E-0046 **Massachusetts General Hospital: Surgical Therapy** An article on the surgical treatment of epilepsy is featured on this Web page. Although it is written in technical terms, patients and their families may still find the article of interest. The article outlines the types of seizures found in patients and emphasizes the importance of presurgical evaluation. Recommendations are made for presurgery diagnostic tests such as neuro-imaging, electroencephalographic testing, neuropsychological testing, and psychosocial assessment. Surgical options for diagnostic tests are also explained. In addition, surgical procedures, and their appropriate application, are described including lesionectomy, temporal resections, extra-temporal resections, and hemispherectomy.
http://neurosurgery.mgh.harvard.edu/ep-sxtre.htm

4E-0047 **New York University, Mount Sinai Comprehensive Epilepsy Center: Surgical Therapy** A guide to surgical therapy for epilepsy is featured on this Web page. The guide addresses who is eligible for surgery and who may benefit the most from surgery. Two main types of surgery are described: resective surgery, which removes the area of the brain causing seizures, and corpus callosotomy, which disconnects the hemispheres of the brain. Risks and outcomes associated with each surgery are described. Tests performed prior to surgery are also described, along with detailed information on the surgical procedures. Costs associated with surgery are briefly addressed.
http://epilepsy.med.nyu.edu/Book/surg.html

VAGAL NERVE STIMULATION

4E-0048 **Epilepsy Foundation: Vagus Nerve Stimulation** A fact sheet on vagus nerve stimulation (VNS) is provided on this Web page. The treatment—designed to be used in addition to medications—is described, along with why it works. Patients who may benefit from VNS, anticipated results, and side effects are also described. http://www.efa.org/answerplace/treatment/vns.html

5.6 WOMEN AND EPILEPSY

4E-0049 **American Family Physician: Pregnancy and Epilepsy** Originally published in the October 1997 issue of *American Family Physician,* this article focuses on epilepsy in pregnancy. The article examines problems associated with epilepsy in pregnancy such as changes in drug metabolism, an increase in seizure frequency, increased risk of fetal bleeding, and a possible decrease in childhood intelligence. Problems associated with antiepileptic drugs are covered, including phenobarbital, valproic acid, carbamazepine, and primidone. Recommendations are made for preconception counseling and pregnancy management. A link at the bottom of the page offers access to a patient information handout on epilepsy in pregnancy. References are also provided.

http://www.aafp.org/afp/971015ap/rochest.html

`4E-0050` **Epilepsy Foundation: Women's Health** Information for women with epilepsy is featured on this Web page. There are fact sheets on menopause and epilepsy, hormones and epilepsy, birth control, and pregnancy. In addition, questions to ask the doctor are provided for common concerns, such as medicine, managing seizures, memory, and pregnancy. Tips for safer living are also featured, including safer bathrooms, kitchens, houses, and kids.

http://www.epilepsyfoundation.org/
answerplace/getsection.cfm?keyname=women

`4E-0051` **Weill Medical College of Cornell University: Pregnancy and Epilepsy** An article on pregnancy and epilepsy is provided on this Web site. The article covers seizure complications during pregnancy, medications, and congenital abnormalities. In addition, breast-feeding, inheritability of the condition, and guidelines for management are included. A bibliography is also found.

http://www.med.cornell.edu/neuro/
patient_care/epilepsy_center/ne-pregnancy.html

5.7 CHILDREN AND EPILEPSY

`4E-0052` **Epilepsy Foundation: Children and Epilepsy** Directed to parents, this site offers comprehensive information on epilepsy in children. Fact sheets examine topics such as the causes of childhood epilepsy, types of seizures, managing seizures, treatment, and finding support. There is also information on antiepileptic medications, the ketogenic diet, surgery, and vagus nerve stimulation. Useful information directed to babysitters and schools is presented, as well as tips for talking to one's doctor and suggestions for safer recreation.

http://www.efa.org/answerplace/getsection.cfm?keyname=parents

`4E-0053` **Epilepsy Ontario: Children Living with Epilepsy** Comprehensive information related to children and epilepsy is featured on this site. Brochures are available online for an overview of epilepsy, treatments for children with epilepsy, diagnostic tests, dealing with doctors who treat epilepsy, related medical conditions, and the psychosocial effects of epilepsy on children. In addition, there is information on stages of childhood development, epilepsy and the

family, and epilepsy and the school setting. Useful fact sheets include a one-page reference for first aid, an information sheet for caregivers, a letter to the child's teacher to explain the condition, and a book list of recommended reading.
http://epilepsyontario.org/faqs/P_T/

5.8 SENIORS AND EPILEPSY

4E-0054 **Epilepsy Foundation: Epilepsy in Later Life** Directed to seniors, this site offers an in-depth article on epilepsy in later life, including treatment, managing seizures, and coping. There is also information on medicines for the elderly and working with the doctor for effective management of the condition.
http://www.efa.org/answerplace/getsection.cfm?keyname=seniors

4E-0055 **Epilepsy Ontario: Seniors and Epilepsy** A series of fact sheets on seniors with epilepsy, for those who are newly diagnosed or who have had the disorder for a long time, is provided on this Web page. Visitors will find information on causes, diagnosis, medications for seizures, mood and perception, stress and coping, and family dynamics. The issue of driving and epilepsy, as well as of menopause and epilepsy, is also addressed.
http://epilepsyontario.org/faqs/seniors/01.html

5.9 CLINICAL TRIALS AND STUDIES

4E-0056 **CenterWatch Clinical Trials Listing Service: Epilepsy** Patients will find clinical trial information for epilepsy on this Web page. The clinical trials are listed by state; hyperlinks lead to further information such as eligibility for the study, its purpose, treatment being tested, and contact information. In addition, the site offers links to research centers specializing in epilepsy and to related Internet links. Visitors can also sign up for an e-mail notification of new clinical trials in epilepsy, as well as newly approved drugs by the Food and Drug Administration (FDA).
http://www.centerwatch.com/patient/studies/cat62.html

4E-0057 **ClinicalTrials.gov** To find clinical trials related to epilepsy, visitors must enter "epilepsy" in the "Search Clinical Trials" tool of this Web site, maintained by the National Institutes of Health. The resulting list of clinical trials contains hyperlinks that offer information on each study such as the sponsor, purpose, a summary of the study, eligibility, location, and contact information.
http://clinicaltrials.gov

6

T O P I C S   A N D   I S S U E S

6.1 Advocacy

4E-0058 | **Citizens United for Research in Epilepsy (CURE)** CURE is a grassroots organization that advocates for more funding for research. The CURE site offers information on research grants, research news, and a short list of links to related sites. There are also brief descriptions of epilepsy and living with epilepsy.
http://www.cureepilepsy.org/

6.2 Clinics and Research Centers

4E-0059 | **Galaxy: Epilepsy Clinics** Epilepsy clinics and medical centers are listed on this Web site. Each link has a brief description of the program. More than 20 programs are found from domestic and international sources.
http://www.galaxy.com/galaxy/Business-and-Commerce/Consumer-Products-and-Services/Health-and-Medicine/Hospitals-Clinics-and-Medical-Centers/Epilepsy-Clinics.html

6.3 Driving with Epilepsy

4E-0060 | **Epilepsy Foundation: Driving and Epilepsy** Resources related to driving and epilepsy are provided on this Web page. Detailed information is provided on driver licensing, reporting requirements for people with epilepsy, and liability issues. There are also tips for safer transportation, along with information on Federal Department of Transportation Regulations and public transportation services.
http://www.efa.org/answerplace/getsection.cfm?keyname=driving

6.4 EMPLOYMENT

4E-0061 **Job Accommodation Network: Epilepsy** A guide to work site accommodations for people with epilepsy is provided on this site. The guide offers employers detailed information on epilepsy, including different types of seizures, photosensitivity, and first aid for seizures. Recommendations for defining an individual's needs are provided. Supplier information is given for accommodations appropriate to photosensitive employees. In addition, there are examples of successful job accommodations. There are also employment resources for people with epilepsy, along with general resources on epilepsy.
http://janweb.icdi.wvu.edu/media/epilepsy.html

6.5 FAMOUS PEOPLE WITH EPILEPSY

4E-0062 **Famous People with Epilepsy** This personal Web page offers a list of famous people with epilepsy, such as Julius Caesar, Napoleon, Vincent van Gogh, Charles Dickens, and Danny Glover. A suggestion form is provided for additions to the list.
http://www.iainmacn.mcmail.com/epilepsy/famous.htm

6.6 FIRST AID AND SAFETY

4E-0063 **Epilepsy Foundation of New Jersey: First Aid for Epilepsy** A brief fact sheet on first aid for epilepsy is offered on this Web page. The fact sheet explains what to do during and after a seizure, as well as when to call a doctor for someone experiencing generalized tonic-clonic seizures. Similar information is provided for complex partial seizures.
http://www.efnj.com/first_aid.shtml

4E-0064 **Epilepsy Foundation: First Aid and Safety** Although this section of the Epilepsy Foundation site is dedicated to teens, the first aid and safety information under the "Seizure Smart Babysitter" section provides useful information for people of all ages. Topics include what seizures look like, simple first aid, and emergency aid. The "Tips for Safer Living" section offers recommendations for safer transportation, recreation, and caring for children.
http://www.epilepsyfoundation.org/
answerplace/getsection.cfm?keyname=teens

6.7 Genetics

4E-0065 **Epilepsy Foundation: Gene Discovery Project** Information on the Epilepsy Foundation's Gene Discovery Project is featured on this site. Patients with epilepsy can fill out a confidential
questionnaire to determine if the epilepsy in their family would be
valuable for further study.
http://www.epilepsyfoundation.org/research/gdp/index.html

4E-0066 **University of Michigan: Epilepsy Genetics News** A news
story, dated March 2000, on the relationship between epilepsy and
genetics is provided on this site. The story describes the findings
of University of Michigan scientists that mutations in a sodium
channel gene may be the cause of one or more types of inherited
epilepsy. A link is provided for the article describing the study in
the April 2000 issue of *Nature Genetics*.
http://www.umich.edu/~newsinfo/Releases/2000/Mar00/r032900b.html

6.8 Historical Perspectives

4E-0067 **World Health Organization (WHO): Historical Overview
of Epilepsy** The World Health Organization offers a historic
overview of epilepsy on this Web page. Information on the condition is presented from as far back as 4500 B.C. The transition from
a spiritual to scientific perspective on the condition is detailed.
http://www.who.int/inf-fs/en/fact168.html

6.9 Legal Rights and Issues

4E-0068 **Epilepsy Foundation of New Jersey: Legal Rights** This
Web site offers a fact sheet on the legal rights of persons with epilepsy. The fact sheet covers topics such as employment, with detailed information on the Americans with Disabilities Act; family
law; criminal justice; driver licensing; education; and health insur-
ance. In addition, treatment for institutionalized patients and Fed-
eral disability benefits are covered. Information on ordering the
124-page booklet entitled *The Legal Rights of Persons with Epilepsy* is provided on the site.
http://www.efnj.com/legal.shtml

4E-0069 **Epilepsy Foundation: Legal Issues** A collection of resources
related to legal rights and issues is presented on this site, created
by the Epilepsy Foundation. Visitors can access information on
driver licensing laws such as reporting requirements, liability, and

licensing issues. In addition, there is information on arrest for seizure-related behavior, epilepsy and violent crime, the armed services, education, child custody, and government assistance.
http://www.epilepsyfoundation.org/
answerplace/getsection.cfm?keyname=legalsystem

6.10 MARKETPLACE

4E-0070 | **Epilepsy Foundation Marketplace** The Epilepsy Foundation Marketplace is an online catalog of books, pamphlets, manuals, and videos related to epilepsy. There are sections of the catalog dedicated to children, employment and legal issues, healthcare professionals, individuals and families, law enforcement, school and recreation, and women. In addition, there is a best-seller section, as well as a section for specialty items such as a pill timer and shirts. All items can be purchased online.
http://www.epilepsyfoundation.org/marketplace/

6.11 RESEARCH INITIATIVES

4E-0071 | **National Institute of Neurological Disorders and Stroke (NINDS): Finding a Cure for Epilepsy** The National Institute of Neurological Disorders and Stroke has posted the results from the "Curing Epilepsy: Focus on the Future" conference of March 2000 on this Web site. At that conference, benchmarks were defined for what it would take to reach a cure for epilepsy. This site outlines the three major initiatives for further research: namely, interrupting and monitoring epileptogenesis, genetic strategies, and developing new therapies.
http://www.ninds.nih.gov/about_ninds/epilepsybenchmarks.htm

6.12 SOCIAL CONSEQUENCES

4E-0072 | **Epilepsy Ontario: Social Relationships** A fact sheet on the importance of social relationships for people with epilepsy is featured on this site. Support groups are emphasized, along with social support for adolescents.
http://epilepsyontario.org/faqs/wellness/soc.html

4E-0073 | **World Health Organization (WHO): Social Consequences and Economic Aspects of Epilepsy** The social consequences for people with epilepsy are examined in this fact sheet, along with economics associated with the disease. The fact sheet notes that fear, misunderstanding, and discrimination are common aspects

of life for people with epilepsy around the world. Legislation and employment are discussed in terms of their discrimination against persons with epilepsy. The financial barriers to treatment, on a global level, are also addressed.
http://www.who.int/inf-fs/en/fact166.html

6.13 STATISTICS

4E-0074 **Centers for Disease Control and Prevention (CDC): Epilepsy Statistics** Statistics on epilepsy are featured on this site, courtesy of the CDC's National Center for Health Statistics. An overview of national statistics is provided, such as the number of Americans with epilepsy, age and region of primary incidence, and the number of visits to a neurologist. Data is also available for download, including epilepsy prevalence sorted by age, sex and age, race and age, family income and age, and geographic region. Related links are provided.
http://www.cdc.gov/nchs/fastats/epilepsy.htm

6.14 SUPPORT GROUPS

4E-0075 **Epilepsy Support Groups** Links to more than 60 epilepsy support groups and organizations from around the world are provided on this Web site, maintained by the University of Washington Regional Epilepsy Center. Most sites are in the United States; however, there are some in Canada, Australia, Europe, Africa, and Asia. http://elliott.hmc.washington.edu/education/support.htm

GLOSSARY

This glossary was created from material drawn from the National Institute of Neurological Disorders and Stroke, as well as suggestions from the editor of this guide, Dr. Gregory Bergey.

absence epilepsy: epilepsy in which the person has repeated absence seizures.

absence seizures: seizures present in absence epilepsy, in which the person experiences a momentary loss of awareness. The person may stare into space for several seconds, be unresponsive, and then return to full awareness. Sometimes there may be associated eye blinks or small muscle twitches.

ACTH (**adrenocorticotropic hormone**): a substance that can be used to treat infantile spasms.

atonic seizures: seizures which cause a sudden loss of muscle tone, also called *drop attacks.*

auras: unusual sensations or movements that warn of an impending, more severe seizure. These auras are actually simple partial seizures in which the person maintains consciousness.

automatisms: strange, repetitious behaviors that occur during a complex partial seizure. Common automatisms may include lip smacking, repetitive swallowing, hand movements, or even walking in circles.

benign epilepsy syndrome: epilepsy syndromes that are not associated with any cognitive or developmental problems. These are often readily controlled and may go into remission. One example is benign rolandic epilepsy of childhood.

benign infantile encephalopathy: a type of epilepsy syndrome that occurs in infants. It is considered benign because it does not seem to impair cognitive functions or development.

benign neonatal convulsions: an epilepsy syndrome in childhood that is now known to involve an abnormality in the potassium ion channel. Dominantly inherited, it is almost universally outgrown in the early months of age and later epilepsy is rare.

biofeedback: a strategy in which individuals learn to control their own brain waves or other normally involuntary functions. This is an experimental treatment for epilepsy.

celiac disease: an intolerance to wheat gluten in foods that can lead to seizures and other symptoms.

clonic seizures: seizures that cause repeated jerking movements of muscles on both sides of the body.

complex partial seizures: seizures that originate from a focal region or a small part of the brain, but have associated alteration of consciousness. Many complex partial seizures originate from the temporal lobes, but this type of seizure can also, less commonly, come from frontal, parietal, or occipital lobe regions. A complex partial seizure can spread to involve both sides of the brain and produce a secondarily generalized tonic-clonic seizure.

convulsions: seizures accompanied by tonic-clonic jerking of all extremities with associated loss of consciousness.

corpus callosotomy: seizure surgery that cuts the band of nerve fibers that connects the right and left hemispheres of the brain. Sometimes only a part of the band is cut. Patients with atonic seizures or drop attacks are the best candidates for this procedure, but unlike other types of seizure surgery, the seizures are rarely totally controlled.

CT (**computed tomography**): a sophisticated type of X-ray that reveals brain structures that cannot be seen with routine X-rays. While CT can reveal many features (normal and abnormal) it is not nearly as sensitive as magnetic resonance imaging (MRI, see below) in the evaluation of a patient with epilepsy.

drop attacks: seizures that cause sudden falls; another term for atonic seizures.

dysplasia: areas of congenitally misplaced or abnormally formed neurons in the brain. While some dysplasias can be the cause of epilepsy, many times they do not cause problems.

early myoclonic encephalopathy: a type of epilepsy syndrome that usually includes neurological and developmental problems.

eclampsia: a life-threatening condition that can develop in pregnant women. Its symptoms include sudden elevations of blood pressure and seizures.

electroencephalogram (EEG): a test that records brain activity (waves) using electrodes placed on the scalp to sample electrical activity (normal and abnormal).

epilepsy syndromes: disorders that include seizure type, EEG pattern, possible genetic factors, other associated conditions, and prognosis.

excitatory neurotransmitters: nerve-signaling chemicals that increase activity in neurons.

febrile seizures: seizures in infants and children that are associated with a high fever.

frontal lobe epilepsy: a type of epilepsy that originates in the frontal lobe of the brain. It usually involves a cluster of short seizures with a sudden onset and termination.

functional MRI (**functional magnetic resonance imaging**): a type of MRI (see below), still being developed, that can sometimes determine functional areas of the brain, for instance the location of speech or motor areas.

GABA (**gamma-aminobutyric acid**): a very important inhibitory neurotransmitter in the brain. Abnormalities in brain GABA and pathways may contribute to some types of epilepsy. Some antiepileptic drugs act by increasing GABA activity in the brain.

generalized seizures: seizures that result from abnormal electrical activity coming from both sides of the brain instead of just one region or focus. Seizures can begin as generalized seizures (primary generalized seizures) or spread from partial seizures to become generalized (secondarily generalized seizures). Most secondarily generalized seizures are tonic-clonic seizures. Examples of primary generalized seizures include absence seizures, tonic seizures, myoclonic seizures, and some tonic-clonic seizures.

glia: cells that regulate concentrations of chemicals that affect neuron signaling and perform other important functions in the brain.

glutamate: an excitatory neurotransmitter that may play a role in some types of epilepsy.

grand mal seizures: an older term for *tonic-clonic seizures.*

hemispheres: the right and left halves of the brain.

hippocampus: a brain structure deep in the temporal lobes important for memory and learning. Temporal lobe complex partial seizures frequently originate in the hippocampus.

idiopathic epilepsy: epilepsy with an unknown cause.

infantile spasms: clusters of seizures that usually begin before the age of six months. During these seizures the infant may bend and cry out.

inhibitory neurotransmitters: chemicals in the brain that signal between nerve cells and decrease activity. GABA (see above) is the most important inhibitory neurotransmitter in the brain.

intractable epilepsy: epilepsy in which a person continues to experience seizures even with the best available treatment.

ion channels: molecular "gates" that control the flow of ions in and out of cells and regulate neuron signaling.

juvenile myoclonic epilepsy (JME): an epilepsy syndrome where the seizures begin in late childhood or adolescence. There are sudden myoclonic jerks, made worse by sleep deprivation. There often are rare associated generalized tonic-clonic seizures and some patients also have absence seizures. Most patients with JME can have their seizures easily controlled with medications.

ketogenic diet: a strict diet, rich in fats and low in carbohydrates that relies on the breakdown of fats for the main energy source. The ketogenic diet is used as a treatment of seizures in children with difficult to control seizures. Although some studies are being performed in adults, the use of this diet in adults is much less well established.

kindling: a phenomenon in which a small stimulus or change in neuronal activity (initially too small to cause a seizure), if repeated, can later trigger an epileptic seizure. Kindling has been demonstrated in animals; it is not known what role it plays in humans.

LaFora's disease: a severe, progressive form of epilepsy that begins in childhood and has been linked to a gene that helps to break down carbohydrates.

Lennox-Gastaut syndrome: an epileptic syndrome that begins in childhood and often includes multiple seizure types and developmental problems. Patients with this syndrome often have difficulty achieving total seizure control.

lesion: a damaged or dysfunctional part of the brain or other part of the body.

lesionectomy: removal of a specific brain lesion.

lobectomy: removal of part of a lobe of a brain, usually to remove the seizure focus and achieve seizure control in patients who cannot have their seizures controlled with medications.

magnetic resonance spectroscopy (MRS): a type of brain imaging that reveals differences and abnormalities in biochemical makeup.

magnetoencephalogram (MEG): a diagnostic recording technique that detects the magnetic signals generated by neurons to allow doctors to monitor brain activity at different points in the brain over time, revealing regions of abnormal electrical activity.

metabolized: broken down or otherwise transformed by the body.

monotherapy: treatment with only one antiepileptic drug.

MRI (magnetic resonance imaging): a type of brain imaging that uses very strong magnetic fields (not X-rays) to reveal detailed images of the structure of the brain and any abnormalities. MRI is much more sensitive than CT in revealing most causes of epilepsy. See also functional MRI.

multiple sub-pial transection: a type of operation in which surgeons make a series of cuts in the brain that are designed to prevent seizures from spreading into other parts of the brain while leaving the person's normal abilities intact. This type of seizure surgery is often used when operating on brain regions important for speech or motor functions.

mutation: an abnormality in a gene.

myoclonic seizures: seizures that cause sudden jerks or twitches, especially in the upper body, arms, or legs.

near-infrared spectroscopy: a technique that can detect oxygen levels in brain tissue.

neurocysticercosis: a parasitic infection of the brain caused by the larvae of the tapeworm. A very common cause of epilepsy in Asia, Central and South America.

neurotransmitters: nerve-signaling chemicals.

nonconvulsive: any type of seizure that does not include violent muscle contractions.

nonepileptic events: any phenomena that look like seizures but which do not include seizure activity in the brain. Nonepileptic events may include psychogenic seizures or symptoms of medical disorders such as sleep disorders, Tourette syndrome, or cardiac arrhythmia.

occipital lobe epilepsy: epilepsy with seizures that originate in the occipital lobe of the brain. It usually begins with visual hallucinations, rapid eye blinking, or other eye-related symptoms.

parietal lobe epilepsy: epilepsy that originates in the parietal lobe of the brain. The symptoms of parietal lobe epilepsy closely resemble those of temporal lobe epilepsy or other syndromes.

partial seizures: seizures originating from a certain region of the brain. The symptoms experienced depend upon the region of brain involved.

PET (positron emission tomography): a type of brain scan that shows normal and abnormal brain metabolism.

petit mal seizures: an older term for *absence seizures.*

photosensitive epilepsy: epilepsy with seizures triggered by flickering or flashing lights. It also may be called photic epilepsy or photogenic epilepsy.

prednisone: a drug that can be used to treat infantile spasms.

progressive epilepsy syndromes: epilepsy syndromes in which seizures and/or the person's cognitive or motor abilities get worse.

progressive myoclonus epilepsies: a group of epilepsy syndromes characterized by increasing, difficult to control seizures (including myoclonic seizures) and worsening neurologic function. One type (Unverricht-Lundborg or Baltic myoclonus) is associated with an abnormality in the gene that codes for cystatin B, a protein that regulates enzymes that break down other proteins.

pseudoseizure: another term for a nonepileptic event.

psychogenic seizure: a type of nonepileptic event that is caused by psychological factors.

psychomotor epilepsy: an older term for complex partial seizures. Often these seizures originate from the temporal lobe. The term psychomotor refers to the unusual sensations, emotions, and behavior seen with these seizures.

Ramsay Hunt syndrome type II: a type of rare and severe progressive epilepsy that usually begins in early adulthood.

Rasmussen's encephalitis: a progressive type of epilepsy in which the focus of epileptic activity expands over time. This type of epilepsy is sometimes treated with hemispherectomy.

seizure focus: an area of the brain where seizures originate.

seizure threshold: a term that refers to a person's susceptibility to seizures.

seizure triggers: phenomena that trigger seizures in some people. Seizure triggers do not cause epilepsy but can lead to first seizures or cause breakthrough seizures in people who otherwise experience good seizure control with their medication.

simple partial seizures: seizures that affect only one part of the brain. People experiencing simple partial seizures remain conscious but may experience unusual feelings or sensations.

SPECT (single photon emission computed tomography): a type of brain scan sometimes used to locate seizure foci in the brain.

status epilepticus: a potentially life-threatening condition in which seizures are prolonged or recur before the person can regain consciousness.

stereotyped: similar every time. In epilepsy this refers to the symptoms an individual person has and to the progression of those symptoms.

sudden unexplained death in epilepsy (SUDEP): death that occurs suddenly for no discernible reason. Epilepsy increases the risk of sudden explained death about two-fold.

temporal lobe epilepsy: the most common epilepsy syndrome with complex partial seizures. Only about 50% of patients with temporal lobe epilepsy can have their seizures controlled with medications.

temporal lobe resection (temporal lobectomy): the most commonly performed seizure surgery. Typically the anterior portion of the temporal lobe is removed along with the deeper structures (i.e. amygdala and hippocampus).

tonic seizures: seizures that cause stiffening of muscles of the body, generally those in the back, legs, and arms.

tonic-clonic seizures: seizures that cause a mixture of symptoms, including loss of consciousness, stiffening of the body, and repeated jerks of the arms and legs. In the past these seizures were sometimes referred to as *grand mal seizures*.

transcranial magnetic stimulation (TMS): a procedure that uses a strong magnet held outside the head to influence brain activity. This is an experimental treatment for seizures.

8

WEB SITE AND
TOPICAL INDEX

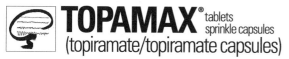

TOPAMAX® tablets sprinkle capsules
(topiramate/topiramate capsules)

Prescribing Information

DESCRIPTION

Topiramate is a sulfamate-substituted monosaccharide that is intended for use as an antiepileptic drug. TOPAMAX® (topiramate) Tablets are available as 25 mg, 100 mg, and 200 mg round tablets for oral administration. TOPAMAX® (topiramate capsules) Sprinkle Capsules are available as 15 mg and 25 mg sprinkle capsules for oral administration as whole capsules or opened and sprinkled onto soft food.

Topiramate is a white crystalline powder with a bitter taste. Topiramate is most soluble in alkaline solutions containing sodium hydroxide or sodium phosphate and having a pH of 9 to 10. It is freely soluble in acetone, chloroform, dimethylsulfoxide, and ethanol. The solubility in water is 9.8 mg/mL. Its saturated solution has a pH of 6.3. Topiramate has the molecular formula $C_{12}H_{21}NO_8S$ and a molecular weight of 339.37. Topiramate is designated chemically as 2,3:4,5-Di-O-isopropylidene-β-D-fructopyranose sulfamate and has the following structural formula:

$$CH_2OSO_2NH_2$$

TOPAMAX® (topiramate) Tablets contain the following inactive ingredients: lactose monohydrate, pregelatinized starch, microcrystalline cellulose, sodium starch glycolate, magnesium stearate, purified water, carnauba wax, hydroxypropyl methylcellulose, titanium dioxide, polyethylene glycol, synthetic iron oxide (100 and 200 mg tablets) and polysorbate 80.

TOPAMAX® (topiramate capsules) Sprinkle Capsules contain topiramate coated beads in a hard gelatin capsule. The inactive ingredients are: sugar spheres (sucrose and starch), povidone, cellulose acetate, gelatin, silicone dioxide, sodium lauryl sulfate, titanium dioxide, and black pharmaceutical ink.

CLINICAL PHARMACOLOGY
Mechanism of Action:

The precise mechanism by which topiramate exerts its antiseizure effect is unknown; however, electrophysiological and biochemical studies of the effects of topiramate on cultured neurons have revealed three properties that may contribute to topiramate's antiepileptic efficacy. First, action potentials elicited repetitively by a sustained depolarization of the neurons are blocked by topiramate in a time-dependent manner, suggestive of a state-dependent sodium channel blocking action. Second, topiramate increases the frequency at which γ-aminobutyrate (GABA) activates $GABA_A$ receptors, and enhances the ability of GABA to induce a flux of chloride ions into neurons, suggesting that topiramate potentiates the activity of this inhibitory neurotransmitter. This effect was not blocked by flumazenil, a benzodiazepine antagonist, nor did topiramate increase the duration of the channel open time, differentiating topiramate from barbiturates that modulate $GABA_A$ receptors. Third, topiramate antagonizes the ability of kainate to activate the kainate/AMPA (α-amino-3-hydroxy-5-methylisoxazole-4-propionic acid; non-NMDA) subtype of excitatory amino acid (glutamate) receptor, but has no apparent effect on the activity of N-methyl-D-aspartate (NMDA) at the NMDA receptor subtype. These effects of topiramate are concentration-dependent within the range of 1 μM to 200 μM.

Topiramate also inhibits some isoenzymes of carbonic anhydrase (CA-II and CA-IV). This pharmacologic effect is generally weaker than that of acetazolamide, a known carbonic anhydrase inhibitor, and is not thought to be a major contributing factor to topiramate's antiepileptic activity.

Pharmacodynamics:

Topiramate has anticonvulsant activity in rat and mouse maximal electroshock seizure (MES) tests. Topiramate is only weakly effective in blocking clonic seizures induced by the $GABA_A$ receptor antagonist, pentylenetetrazole. Topiramate is also effective in rodent models of epilepsy, which include tonic and absence-like seizures in the spontaneous epileptic rat (SER) and tonic and clonic seizures induced in rats by kindling of the amygdala or by global ischemia.

Pharmacokinetics:

The sprinkle formulation is bioequivalent to the immediate release tablet formulation and, therefore, may be substituted as a therapeutic equivalent.

Absorption of topiramate is rapid, with peak plasma concentrations occurring at approximately 2 hours following a 400 mg oral dose. The relative bioavailability of topiramate from the tablet formulation is about 80% compared to a solution. The bioavailability of topiramate is not affected by food.

The pharmacokinetics of topiramate are linear with dose proportional increases in plasma concentration over the dose range studied (200 to 800 mg/day). The mean plasma elimination half-life is 21 hours after single or multiple doses. Steady state is thus reached in about 4 days in patients with normal renal function. Topiramate is 13-17% bound to human plasma proteins over the concentration range of 1-250 μg/mL.

Metabolism and Excretion:

Topiramate is not extensively metabolized and is primarily eliminated unchanged in the urine (approximately 70% of an administered dose). Six metabolites have been identified in humans, none of which constitutes more than 5% of an administered dose. The metabolites are formed via hydroxylation, hydrolysis, and glucuronidation. There is evidence of renal tubular reabsorption of topiramate. In rats, given probenecid to inhibit tubular reabsorption, along with topiramate, a significant increase in renal clearance of topiramate was observed. This interaction has not been evaluated in humans. Overall, oral plasma clearance (CL/F) is approximately 20 to 30 mL/min in humans following oral administration.

Pharmacokinetic Interactions (see also Drug Interactions):

Antiepileptic Drugs

Potential interactions between topiramate and standard AEDs were assessed in controlled clinical pharmacokinetic studies in patients with epilepsy. The effect of these interactions on mean plasma AUCs are summarized under **PRECAUTIONS (Table 3)**.

Special Populations:
Renal Impairment:

The clearance of topiramate was reduced by 42% in moderately renally impaired (creatinine clearance 30-69 mL/min/1.73m²) and by 54% in severely renally impaired subjects (creatinine clearance <30 mL/min/1.73m²) compared to normal renal function subjects (creatinine clearance >70 mL/min/1.73m²). Since topiramate is presumed to undergo significant tubular reabsorption, it is uncertain whether this experience can be generalized to all situations of renal impairment. It is conceivable that some forms of renal disease could differentially affect glomerular filtration rate and tubular reabsorption resulting in a clearance of topiramate not predicted by creatinine clearance. In general, however, use of one-half the usual dose is recommended in patients with moderate or severe renal impairment.

Hemodialysis:

Topiramate is cleared by hemodialysis. Using a high efficiency, counterflow, single pass-dialysate hemodialysis procedure, topiramate dialysis clearance was 120 mL/min with blood flow through the dialyzer at 400 mL/min. This high clearance (compared to 20-30 mL/min total oral clearance in healthy adults) will remove a clinically significant amount of topiramate from the patient over the hemodialysis treatment period. Therefore, a supplemental dose may be required (see **DOSAGE AND ADMINISTRATION**).

Hepatic Impairment:

In hepatically impaired subjects, the clearance of topiramate may be decreased; the mechanism underlying the decrease is not well understood.

Age, Gender, and Race:

Clearance of topiramate in adults was not affected by age (18-67 years), gender, or race.

Pediatric Pharmacokinetics:

Pharmacokinetics of topiramate were evaluated in patients ages 4 to 17 years receiving one or two other antiepileptic drugs. Pharmacokinetic profiles were obtained after one week at doses of 1, 3, and 9 mg/kg/day. Clearance was independent of dose.

Pediatric patients have a 50% higher clearance and consequently shorter elimination half-life than adults. Consequently, the plasma concentration for the same mg/kg dose may be lower in pediatric patients compared to adults. As in adults, hepatic enzyme-inducing antiepileptic drugs decrease the steady state plasma concentrations of topiramate.

CLINICAL STUDIES

The results of controlled clinical trials established the efficacy of TOPAMAX® (topiramate) as adjunctive therapy in adults and pediatric patients ages 2-16 years with partial onset seizures or primary generalized tonic-clonic seizures, and in patients 2 years of age and older with seizures associated with Lennox-Gastaut syndrome.

The studies described in the following sections were conducted using TOPAMAX® (topiramate) Tablets.

Controlled Trials in Patients With Partial Onset Seizures
Adults With Partial Onset Seizures
The effectiveness of topiramate as an adjunctive treatment for adults with partial onset seizures was established in five multicenter, randomized, double-blind, placebo-controlled trials, two comparing several dosages of topiramate and placebo and three comparing a single dosage with placebo, in patients with a history of partial onset seizures, with or without secondarily generalized seizures.

Patients in these studies were permitted a maximum of two antiepileptic drugs (AEDs) in addition to TOPAMAX® Tablets or placebo. In each study, patients were stabilized on optimum dosages of their concomitant AEDs during an 8-12 week baseline phase. Patients who experienced at least 12 (or 8, for 8-week baseline studies) partial onset seizures, with or without secondary generalization, during the baseline phase were randomly assigned to placebo or a specified dose of TOPAMAX® Tablets in addition to their other AEDs.

Following randomization, patients began the double-blind phase of treatment. Patients received active drug beginning at 100 mg per day; the dose was then increased by 100 mg or 200 mg/day increments weekly or every other week until the assigned dose was reached, unless intolerance prevented increases. After titration, patients entered an 8- or 12-week stabilization period. The numbers of patients randomized to each dose, and the actual mean, and median doses in the stabilization period are shown in Table 1.

Pediatric Patients Ages 2-16 Years With Partial Onset Seizures
The effectiveness of topiramate as an adjunctive treatment for pediatric patients ages 2-16 years with partial onset seizures was established in a multicenter, randomized, double-blind, placebo-controlled trial, comparing topiramate and placebo in patients with a history of partial onset seizures, with or without secondarily generalized seizures.

Patients in this study were permitted a maximum of two antiepileptic drugs (AEDs) in addition to TOPAMAX® Tablets or placebo. In this study, patients were stabilized on optimum dosages of their concomitant AEDs during an 8-week baseline phase. Patients who experienced at least six partial onset seizures, with or without secondarily generalized seizures, during the baseline phase were randomly assigned to placebo or TOPAMAX® Tablets in addition to their other AEDs.

Following randomization, patients began the double-blind phase of treatment. Patients received active drug beginning at 25 or 50 mg per day; the dose was then increased by 25 mg to 150 mg/day increments every other week until the assigned dosage of 125, 175, 225, or 400 mg/day based on patients' weight to approximate a dosage of 6 mg/kg per day was reached, unless intolerance prevented increases. After titration, patients entered an 8-week stabilization period.

Controlled Trials in Patients With Primary Generalized Tonic-Clonic Seizures
The effectiveness of topiramate as an adjunctive treatment for primary generalized tonic-clonic seizures in patients 2 years old and older was established in a multicenter, randomized, double-blind, placebo-controlled trial, comparing a single dosage of topiramate and placebo.

Patients in this study were permitted a maximum of two antiepileptic drugs (AEDs) in addition to TOPAMAX® or placebo. Patients were stabilized on optimum dosages of their concomitant AEDs during an 8-week baseline phase. Patients who experienced at least three primary generalized tonic-clonic seizures during the baseline phase were randomly assigned to placebo or TOPAMAX® in addition to their other AEDs. Following randomization, patients began the double-blind phase of treatment. Patients received active drug beginning at 50 mg per day for four weeks; the dose was then increased by 50 mg to 150 mg/day increments every other week until the assigned dose of 175, 225, or 400 mg/day based on patients' body weight to approximate a dosage of 6 mg/kg per day was reached, unless intolerance prevented increases. After titration, patients entered a 12-week stabilization period.

Controlled Trial in Patients With Lennox-Gastaut Syndrome
The effectiveness of topiramate as an adjunctive treatment for seizures associated with Lennox-Gastaut syndrome was established in a multicenter, randomized, double-blind, placebo-controlled trial comparing a single dosage of topiramate with placebo in patients 2 years of age and older.

Patients in this study were permitted a maximum of two antiepileptic drugs (AEDs) in addition to TOPAMAX® or placebo. Patients who were experiencing at least 60 seizures per month before study entry were stabilized on optimum dosages of their concomitant AEDs during a four week baseline phase. Following baseline, patients were randomly assigned to placebo or TOPAMAX® in addition to their other AEDs. Active drug was titrated beginning at 1 mg/kg per day for a week; the dose was then increased to 3 mg/kg per day for one week then to 6 mg/kg per day. After titration, patients entered an 8-week stabilization period. The primary measures of effectiveness were the percent reduction in drop attacks and a parental global rating of seizure severity.

Table 1: Topiramate Dose Summary During the Stabilization Periods of Each of Five Double-Blind, Placebo-Controlled, Add-On Trials in Adults with Partial Onset Seizures[b]

| Protocol | Stabilization Dose | Placebo[a] | Target Topiramate Dosage (mg/day) | | | | |
			200	400	600	800	1,000
YD	N	42	42	40	41	–	–
	Mean Dose	5.9	200	390	556	–	–
	Median Dose	6.0	200	400	600	–	–
YE	N	44	–	–	40	45	40
	Mean Dose	9.7	–	–	544	739	796
	Median Dose	10.0	–	–	600	800	1,000
Y1	N	23	–	19	–	–	–
	Mean Dose	3.8	–	395	–	–	–
	Median Dose	4.0	–	400	–	–	–
Y2	N	30	–	–	28	–	–
	Mean Dose	5.7	–	–	522	–	–
	Median Dose	6.0	–	–	600	–	–
Y3	N	28	–	–	–	25	–
	Mean Dose	7.9	–	–	–	568	–
	Median Dose	8.0	–	–	–	600	–

[a] Placebo dosages are given as the number of tablets. Placebo target dosages were as follows: Protocol Y1, 4 tablets/day; Protocols YD and Y2, 6 tablets/day; Protocol Y3, 8 tablets/day; Protocol YE, 10 tablets/day.
[b] Dose-response studies were not conducted for other indications or pediatric partial onset seizures.

In all add-on trials, the reduction in seizure rate from baseline during the entire double-blind phase was measured. The median percent reductions in seizure rates and the responder rates (fraction of patients with at least a 50% reduction) by treatment group for each study are shown below in Table 2. As described above, a global improvement in seizure severity was also assessed in the Lennox-Gastaut trial.

Table 2: Efficacy Results in Double-Blind, Placebo-Controlled, Add-On Trials

| Protocol | Efficacy Results | Placebo | Target Topiramate Dosage (mg/day) | | | | | |
			200	400	600	800	1,000	≈6 mg/kg/day*
Partial Onset Seizures Studies in Adults								
YD	N	45	45	45	46	–	–	–
	Median % Reduction	11.6	27.2[a]	47.5[b]	44.7[c]	–	–	–
	% Responders	18	24	44[d]	46[d]	–	–	–
YE	N	47	–	–	48	48	47	–
	Median % Reduction	1.7	–	–	40.8[c]	41.0[c]	36.0[c]	–
	% Responders	9	–	–	40[c]	41[c]	36[d]	–
Y1	N	24	–	23	–	–	–	–
	Median % Reduction	1.1	–	40.7[e]	–	–	–	–
	% Responders	8	–	35[d]	–	–	–	–
Y2	N	30	–	–	30	–	–	–
	Median % Reduction	-12.2	–	–	46.4[f]	–	–	–
	% Responders	10	–	–	47[c]	–	–	–
Y3	N	28	–	–	–	28	–	–
	Median % Reduction	-20.6	–	–	–	24.3[c]	–	–
	% Responders	0	–	–	–	43[c]	–	–

Studies in Pediatric Patients

YP	N	45	–	–	–	–	–	41
	Median % Reduction	10.5	–	–	–	–	–	33.1[d]
	% Responders	20	–	–	–	–	–	39
Primary Generalized Tonic-Clonic[h]								
YTC	N	40	–	–	–	–	–	39
	Median % Reduction	9.0	–	–	–	–	–	56.7[d]
	% Responders	20	–	–	–	–	–	56[c]
Lennox-Gastaut Syndrome[i]								
YL	N	49	–	–	–	–	–	46
	Median % Reduction	-5.1	–	–	–	–	–	14.8[d]
	% Responders	14	–	–	–	–	–	28[g]
	Improvement in Seizure Severity[j]	28	–	–	–	–	–	52[d]

Comparisons with placebo: [a] p=0.080; [b] p≤0.010; [c] p≤0.001; [d] p≤0.050; [e] p=0.065; [f] p≤0.005; [g] p=0.071; [h] Median % reduction and % responders are reported for PGTC Seizures; [i] Median % reduction and % responders for drop attacks, i.e., toxic or atonic seizures; [j] Percent of subjects who were minimally, much, or very much improved from baseline

* For Protocols YP and YTC, protocol-specified target dosages (<9.3 mg/kg/day) were assigned based on subject's weight to approximate a dosage of 6 mg/kg per day; these dosages corresponded to mg/day dosages of 125, 175, 225, and 400 mg/day.

Subset analyses of the antiepileptic efficacy of TOPAMAX® Tablets in these studies showed no differences as a function of gender, race, age, baseline seizure rate, or concomitant AED.

INDICATIONS AND USAGE

TOPAMAX® (topiramate) Tablets and TOPAMAX® (topiramate capsules) Sprinkle Capsules are indicated as adjunctive therapy for adults and pediatric patients ages 2-16 years with partial onset seizures, or primary generalized tonic-clonic seizures, and in patients 2 years of age and older with seizures associated with Lennox-Gastaut syndrome.

CONTRAINDICATIONS

TOPAMAX® is contraindicated in patients with a history of hypersensitivity to any component of this product.

WARNINGS

Acute Myopia and Secondary Angle Closure Glaucoma

A syndrome consisting of acute myopia associated with secondary angle closure glaucoma has been reported in patients receiving TOPAMAX®. Symptoms include acute onset of decreased visual acuity and/or ocular pain. Opthalmologic findings can include myopia, anterior chamber shallowing, ocular hyperemia (redness) and increased intraocular pressure. Mydriasis may or may not be present. This syndrome may be associated with supraciliary effusion resulting in anterior displacement of the lens and iris, with secondary angle closure glaucoma. Symptoms typically occur within 1 month of initiating TOPAMAX® therapy. In contrast to primary narrow angle glaucoma, which is rare under 40 years of age, secondary angle closure glaucoma associated with topiramate has been reported in pediatric patients as well as adults. The primary treatment to reverse symptoms is discontinuation of TOPAMAX® as rapidly as possible, according to the judgement of the treating physician. Other measures, in conjunction with discontinuation of TOPAMAX®, may be helpful.

Elevated intraocular pressure of any etiology, if left untreated, can lead to serious sequelae including permanent vision loss.

Withdrawal of AEDs

Antiepileptic drugs, including TOPAMAX®, should be withdrawn gradually to minimize the potential of increased seizure frequency.

Cognitive/Neuropsychiatric Adverse Events

Adults

Adverse events most often associated with the use of TOPAMAX® were central nervous system related. In adults, the most significant of these can be classified into two general categories: 1) psychomotor slowing, difficulty with concentration, and speech or language problems, in particular, word-finding difficulties and 2) somnolence or fatigue. Additional nonspecific CNS effects occasionally observed with topiramate as add-on therapy include dizziness or imbalance, confusion, memory problems, and exacerbation of mood disturbances (e.g., irritability and depression).

Reports of psychomotor slowing, speech and language problems, and difficulty with concentration and attention were common in adults. Although in some cases these events were mild to moderate, they at times led to withdrawal from treatment. The incidence of psychomotor slowing is only marginally dose-related, but both language problems and difficulty with concentration or attention clearly increased in frequency with increasing dosage in the five double-blind trials [see **ADVERSE REACTIONS, Table 5**].

Somnolence and fatigue were the most frequently reported adverse events during clinical trials with TOPAMAX®. These events were generally mild to moderate and occurred early in therapy. While the incidence of somnolence does not appear to be dose-related, that of fatigue increases at dosages above 400 mg/day.

Pediatric Patients

In double-blind clinical studies, the incidences of cognitive/neuropsychiatric adverse events in pediatric patients were generally lower than previously observed in adults. These events included psychomotor slowing, difficulty with concentration/attention, speech disorders/related speech problems and language problems. The most frequently reported neuropsychiatric events in this population were somnolence and fatigue. No patients discontinued treatment due to adverse events in double-blind trials.

Sudden Unexplained Death in Epilepsy (SUDEP)

During the course of premarketing development of TOPAMAX® (topiramate) Tablets, 10 sudden and unexplained deaths were recorded among a cohort of treated patients (2,796 subject years of exposure). This represents an incidence of 0.0035 deaths per patient year. Although this rate exceeds that expected in a healthy population matched for age and sex, it is within the range of estimates for the incidence of sudden unexplained deaths in patients with epilepsy not receiving TOPAMAX® (ranging from 0.0005 for the general population of patients with epilepsy, to 0.003 for a clinical trial population similar to that in the TOPAMAX® program, to 0.005 for patients with refractory epilepsy).

PRECAUTIONS

General:

Kidney Stones

A total of 32/2,086 (1.5%) of adults exposed to topiramate during its development reported the occurrence of kidney stones, an incidence about 2-4 times that expected in a similar, untreated population. As in the general population, the incidence of stone formation among topiramate treated patients was higher in men. Kidney stones have also been reported in pediatric patients.

An explanation for the association of TOPAMAX® and kidney stones may lie in the fact that topiramate is a weak carbonic anhydrase inhibitor. Carbonic anhydrase inhibitors, e.g., acetazolamide or dichlorphenamide, promote stone formation by reducing urinary citrate excretion and by increasing urinary pH. The concomitant use of TOPAMAX® with other carbonic anhydrase inhibitors or potentially in patients on a ketogenic diet may create a physiological environment that increases the risk of kidney stone formation, and should therefore be avoided.

Increased fluid intake increases the urinary output, lowering the concentration of substances involved in stone formation. Hydration is recommended to reduce new stone formation.

Paresthesia

Paresthesia, an effect associated with the use of other carbonic anhydrase inhibitors, appears to be a common effect of TOPAMAX.®

Adjustment of Dose in Renal Failure

The major route of elimination of unchanged topiramate and its metabolites is via the kidney. Dosage adjustment may be required (see **DOSAGE AND ADMINISTRATION**).

Decreased Hepatic Function

In hepatically impaired patients, topiramate should be administered with caution as the clearance of topiramate may be decreased.

Information for Patients

Patients taking TOPAMAX® should be told to seek immediate medical attention if they experience blurred vision or periorbital pain.

Patients, particularly those with predisposing factors, should be instructed to maintain an adequate fluid intake in order to minimize the risk of renal stone formation [see **PRECAUTIONS: General**, for support regarding hydration as a preventative measure].

Patients should be warned about the potential for somnolence, dizziness, confusion, and difficulty concentrating and advised not to drive or operate machinery until they have gained sufficient experience on topiramate to gauge whether it adversely affects their mental and/or motor performance.

Additional food intake may be considered if the patient is losing weight while on this medication.

Please refer to the end of the product labeling for important information on how to take TOPAMAX® (topiramate capsules) Sprinkle Capsules.

Drug Interactions:

Antiepileptic Drugs

Potential interactions between topiramate and standard AEDs were assessed in controlled clinical pharmacokinetic studies in patients with epilepsy. The effects of these interactions on mean plasma AUCs are summarized in the following table:

In Table 3, the second column (AED concentration) describes what happens to the concentration of the AED listed in the first column when topiramate is added.

The third column (topiramate concentration) describes how the coadministration of a drug listed in the first column modifies the concentration of topiramate in experimental settings when TOPAMAX® was given alone.

Table 3: Summary of AED Interactions with TOPAMAX®

AED Co-administered	AED Concentration	Topiramate Concentration
Phenytoin	NC or 25% increase[a]	48% decrease
Carbamazepine (CBZ)	NC	40% decrease
CBZ epoxide[b]	NC	NE
Valproic acid	11% decrease	14% decrease
Phenobarbital	NC	NE
Primidone	NC	NE

[a] = Plasma concentration increased 25% in some patients, generally those on a b.i.d. dosing regimen of phenytoin.
[b] = is not administered but is an active metabolite of carbamazepine.
NC = Less than 10% change in plasma concentration.
AED = Antiepileptic drug.
NE = Not Evaluated.

Other Drug Interactions

Digoxin: In a single-dose study, serum digoxin AUC was decreased by 12% with concomitant TOPAMAX® administration. The clinical relevance of this observation has not been established.

CNS Depressants: Concomitant administration of TOPAMAX® and alcohol or other CNS depressant drugs has not been evaluated in clinical studies. Because of the potential of topiramate to cause CNS depression, as well as other cognitive and/or neuropsychiatric adverse events, topiramate should be used with extreme caution if used in combination with alcohol and other CNS depressants.

Oral Contraceptives: In a pharmacokinetic interaction study with oral contraceptives using a combination product containing norethindrone and ethinyl estradiol, TOPAMAX® did not significantly affect the clearance of norethindrone. The mean oral clearance of ethinyl estradiol at 800 mg/day dose was increased by 47% (range: 13-107%). The mean total exposure to the estrogenic component decreased by 18%, 21%, and 30% at daily doses of 200, 400, and 800 mg/day, respectively. Therefore, efficacy of oral contraceptives may be compromised by topiramate. Patients taking oral contraceptives should be asked to report any change in their bleeding patterns. The effect of oral contraceptives on the pharmacokinetics of topiramate is not known.

Others: Concomitant use of TOPAMAX®, a weak carbonic anhydrase inhibitor, with other carbonic anhydrase inhibitors, e.g., acetazolamide or dichlorphenamide, may create a physiological environment that increases the risk of renal stone formation, and should therefore be avoided.

Laboratory Tests: There are no known interactions of topiramate with commonly used laboratory tests.

Carcinogenesis, Mutagenesis, Impairment of Fertility:

An increase in urinary bladder tumors was observed in mice given topiramate (20, 75, and 300 mg/kg) in the diet for 21 months. The elevated bladder tumor incidence, which was statistically significant in males and females receiving 300 mg/kg, was primarily due to the increased occurrence of a smooth muscle tumor considered histomorphologically unique to mice. Plasma exposures in mice receiving 300 mg/kg were approximately 0.5 to 1 times steady state exposures measured in patients receiving topiramate monotherapy at the recommended human dose (RHD) of 400 mg, and 1.5 to 2 times steady state topiramate exposures in patients receiving 400 mg of topiramate plus phenytoin. The relevance of this finding to human carcinogenic risk is uncertain. No evidence of carcinogenicity was seen in rats following oral administration of topiramate for 2 years at doses up to 120 mg/kg (approximately 3 times the RHD on a mg/m^2 basis).

Topiramate did not demonstrate genotoxic potential when tested in a battery of *in vitro* and *in vivo* assays. Topiramate was not mutagenic in the Ames test or the *in vitro* mouse lymphoma assay; it did not increase unscheduled DNA synthesis in rat hepatocytes *in vitro*; and it did not increase chromosomal aberrations in human lymphocytes *in vitro* or in rat bone marrow *in vivo*.

No adverse effects on male or female fertility were observed in rats at doses up to 100 mg/kg (2.5 times the RHD on a mg/m^2 basis).

Pregnancy: Pregnancy Category C.

Topiramate has demonstrated selective developmental toxicity, including teratogenicity, in experimental animal studies. When oral doses of 20, 100, or 500 mg/kg were administered to pregnant mice during the period of organogenesis, the incidence of fetal malformations (primarily craniofacial defects) was increased at all doses. The low dose is approximately 0.2 times the recommended human dose (RHD=400 mg/day) on a mg/m^2 basis. Fetal body weights and skeletal ossification were reduced at 500 mg/kg in conjunction with decreased maternal body weight gain.

In rat studies (oral doses of 20, 100, and 500 mg/kg or 0.2, 2.5, 30 and 400 mg/kg), the frequency of limb malformations (ectrodactyly, micromelia, and amelia) was increased among the offspring of dams treated with 400 mg/kg (10 times the RHD on a mg/m^2 basis) or greater during the organogenesis period of pregnancy. Embryotoxicity (reduced fetal body weights, increased incidence of structural variations) was observed at doses as low as 20 mg/kg (0.5 times the RHD on a mg/m^2 basis). Clinical signs of maternal toxicity were seen at 400 mg/kg and above, and maternal body weight gain was reduced during treatment with 100 mg/kg or greater.

In rabbit studies (20, 60, and 180 mg/kg or 10, 35, and 120 mg/kg orally during organogenesis), embryo/fetal mortality was increased at 35 mg/kg (2 times the RHD on a mg/m^2 basis) or greater, and teratogenic effects (primarily rib and vertebral malformations) were observed at 120 mg/kg (6 times the RHD on a mg/m^2 basis). Evidence of maternal toxicity (decreased body weight gain, clinical signs, and/or mortality) was seen at 35 mg/kg and above.

When female rats were treated during the latter part of gestation and throughout lactation (0.2, 4, 20, and 100 mg/kg or 2, 20, and 200 mg/kg), offspring exhibited decreased viability and delayed physical development at 200 mg/kg (5 times the RHD on a mg/m^2 basis) and reductions in pre- and/or postweaning body weight gain at 2 mg/kg (0.05 times the RHD on a mg/m^2 basis) and above. Maternal toxicity (decreased body weight gain, clinical signs) was evident at 100 mg/kg or greater.

In a rat embryo/fetal development study with a postnatal component (0.2, 2.5, 30 or 400 mg/kg during organogenesis; noted above), pups exhibited delayed physical development at 400 mg/kg (10 times the RHD on a mg/m^2 basis) and persistent reductions in body weight gain at 30 mg/kg (1 times the RHD on a mg/m^2 basis) and higher.

There are no studies using TOPAMAX® in pregnant women. TOPAMAX® should be used during pregnancy only if the potential benefit outweighs the potential risk to the fetus.

In post-marketing experience, cases of hypospadias have been reported in male infants exposed in utero to topiramate, with or without other anticonvulsants; however, a causal relationship with topiramate has not been established.

Labor and Delivery:

In studies of rats where dams were allowed to deliver pups naturally, no drug-related effects on gestation length or parturition were observed at dosage levels up to 200 mg/kg/day.

The effect of TOPAMAX® on labor and delivery in humans is unknown.

Nursing Mothers:

Topiramate is excreted in the milk of lactating rats. It is not known if topiramate is excreted in human milk. Since many drugs are excreted in human milk, and because the potential for serious adverse reactions in nursing infants to TOPAMAX® is unknown, the potential benefit to the mother should be weighed against the potential risk to the infant when considering recommendations regarding nursing.

Pediatric Use:

Safety and effectiveness in patients below the age of 2 years have not been established.

Geriatric Use:

In clinical trials, 2% of patients were over 60. No age related difference in effectiveness or adverse effects were seen. There were no pharmacokinetic differences related to age alone, although the possibility of age-associated renal functional abnormalities should be considered.

Race and Gender Effects:

Evaluation of effectiveness and safety in clinical trials has shown no race or gender related effects.

ADVERSE REACTIONS

The data described in the following section were obtained using TOPAMAX® (topiramate) Tablets.

The most commonly observed adverse events associated with the use of topiramate at dosages of 200 to 400 mg/day in controlled trials in adults with partial onset seizures, primary generalized tonic-clonic seizures, or Lennox-Gastaut syndrome, that were seen at greater frequency in topiramate-treated patients and did not appear to be dose-related were: somnolence, dizziness, ataxia, speech disorders and related speech problems, psychomotor slowing, abnormal vision, difficulty with memory, paresthesia and diplopia [see Table 4]. The most common dose-related adverse events at dosages of 200 to 1,000 mg/day were: fatigue, nervousness, difficulty with concentration or attention, confusion, depression, anorexia, language problems, anxiety, mood problems, and weight decrease [see Table 5].

Adverse events associated with the use of topiramate at dosages of 5 to 9 mg/kg/day in controlled trials in pediatric patients with partial onset seizures, primary generalized tonic-clonic seizures, or Lennox-Gastaut syndrome, that were seen at greater frequency in topiramate-treated patients were: fatigue, somnolence, anorexia, nervousness, difficulty with concentration/attention, difficulty with memory, aggressive reaction, and weight decrease [see Table 6].

In controlled clinical trials in adults, 11% of patients receiving topiramate 200 to 400 mg/day as adjunctive therapy discontinued due to adverse events. This rate appeared to increase at dosages above 400 mg/day. Adverse events associated with discontinuing therapy included somnolence, dizziness, anxiety, difficulty with concentration or attention, fatigue, and paresthesia and increased at dosages above 400 mg/day. None of the pediatric patients who received topiramate adjunctive therapy at 5 to 9 mg/kg/day in controlled clinical trials discontinued due to adverse events.

Approximately 28% of the 1,757 adults with epilepsy who received topiramate at dosages of 200 to 1,600 mg/day in clinical studies discontinued treatment because of adverse events; an individual patient could have reported more than one adverse event. These adverse events were: psychomotor slowing (4.0%), difficulty with memory (3.2%), fatigue (3.2%), confusion (3.1%), somnolence (3.2%), difficulty with concentration/attention (2.9%), anorexia (2.7%), depression (2.6%), dizziness (2.5%), weight decrease (2.5%), nervousness (2.3%), ataxia (2.1%), and paresthesia (2.0%). Approximately 11% of the 310 pediatric patients who received topiramate at dosages up to 30 mg/kg/day discontinued due to adverse events. Adverse events associated with discontinuing therapy included aggravated convulsions (2.3%), difficulty with concentration/attention (1.6%), language problems (1.3%), personality disorder (1.3%), and somnolence (1.3%).

Incidence in Controlled Clinical Trials – Add-On Therapy

Table 4 lists treatment-emergent adverse events that occurred in at least 1% of adults treated with 200 to 400 mg/day topiramate in controlled trials that were numerically more common at this dose than in the patients treated with placebo. In general, most patients who experienced adverse events during the first eight weeks of these trials no longer experienced them by their last visit. Table 6 lists treatment-emergent adverse events that occurred in at least 1% of pediatric patients treated with 5 to 9 mg/kg topiramate in controlled trials that were numerically more common than in patients treated with placebo.

The prescriber should be aware that these data were obtained when TOPAMAX® was added to concurrent antiepileptic drug therapy and cannot be used to predict the frequency of adverse events in the course of usual medical practice where patient characteristics and other factors may differ from those prevailing during clinical studies. Similarly, the cited frequencies cannot be directly compared with data obtained from other clinical investigations involving different treatments, uses, or investigators. Inspection of these frequencies, however, does provide the prescribing physician with a basis to estimate the relative contribution of drug and non-drug factors to the adverse event incidences in the population studied.

Table 4: Incidence of Treatment-Emergent Adverse Events in Placebo-Controlled, Add-On Trials in Adults[a,b]
Where Rate Was > 1% in Either Topiramate Group and Greater Than the Rate in Placebo-Treated Patients

Body System/ Adverse Event [c]	Placebo (N=291)	TOPAMAX® Dosage (mg/day)	
		200-400 (N=183)	600-1,000 (N=414)
Body as a Whole –			
General Disorders			
Fatigue	13	15	30
Asthenia	1	6	3
Back Pain	4	5	3
Chest Pain	3	4	2
Influenza-Like Symptoms	2	3	4
Leg Pain	2	2	4
Hot Flushes	1	2	1
Allergy	1	2	3
Edema	1	2	1
Body Odor	0	1	0
Rigors	0	1	<1
Central & Peripheral Nervous System Disorders			
Dizziness	15	25	32
Ataxia	7	16	14
Speech Disorders/ Related Speech Problems	2	13	11
Paresthesia	4	11	19
Nystagmus	7	10	11
Tremor	6	9	9
Language Problems	1	6	10
Coordination Abnormal	2	4	4
Hypoaesthesia	1	2	1
Gait Abnormal	1	3	2
Muscle Contractions Involuntary	1	2	2
Stupor	0	2	1
Vertigo	1	1	2
Gastro-Intestinal System Disorders			
Nausea	8	10	12
Dyspepsia	6	7	6
Abdominal Pain	4	6	7
Constipation	2	4	3
Gastroenteritis	1	2	1
Dry Mouth	1	2	4
Gingivitis	<1	1	1
GI Disorder	<1	1	0
Hearing and Vestibular Disorders			
Hearing Decreased	1	2	1
Metabolic and Nutritional Disorders			
Weight Decrease	3	9	13
Muscle-Skeletal System Disorders			
Myalgia	1	2	2
Skeletal Pain	0	1	0
Platelet, Bleeding & Clotting Disorders			
Epistaxis	1	2	1
Psychiatric Disorders			
Somnolence	12	29	28
Nervousness	6	16	19
Psychomotor Slowing	2	13	21
Difficulty with Memory	3	12	14
Anorexia	4	10	12
Confusion	5	11	14
Depression	5	5	13
Difficulty with Concentration/ Attention	2	6	14
Mood Problems	2	4	9
Agitation	2	3	3
Aggressive Reaction	2	3	3

Emotional Lability	1	3	3
Cognitive Problems	1	3	3
Libido Decreased	1	2	<1
Apathy	1	1	3
Depersonalization	1	1	2
Reproductive Disorders, Female			
Breast Pain	2	4	0
Amenorrhea	1	2	2
Menorrhagia	0	2	1
Menstrual Disorder	1	2	1
Reproductive Disorders, Male			
Prostatic Disorder	<1	2	0
Resistance Mechanism Disorders			
Infection	1	2	1
Infection Viral	1	2	<1
Moniliasis	<1	1	0
Respiratory System Disorders			
Pharyngitis	2	6	3
Rhinitis	6	7	6
Sinusitis	4	5	6
Dyspnea	1	1	2
Skin and Appendages Disorders			
Skin Disorder	<1	2	1
Sweating Increased	<1	1	<1
Rash Erythematous	<1	1	<1
Special Sense Other, Disorders			
Taste Perversion	0	2	4
Urinary System Disorders			
Hematuria	1	2	<1
Urinary Tract Infection	1	2	3
Micturition Frequency	1	1	2
Urinary Incontinence	<1	2	1
Urine Abnormal	0	1	<1
Vision Disorders			
Vision Abnormal	2	13	10
Diplopia	5	10	10
White Cell and RES Disorders			
Leukopenia	1	2	1

[a] Patients in these add-on trials were receiving 1 to 2 concomitant antiepileptic drugs in addition to TOPAMAX® or placebo.
[b] Values represent the percentage of patients reporting a given adverse event. Patients may have reported more than one adverse event during the study and can be included in more than one adverse event category.
[c] Adverse events reported by at least 1% of patients in the TOPAMAX® 200-400 mg/day group and more common than in the placebo group are listed in this table.

Table 5: Incidence (%) of Dose-Related Adverse Events From Placebo-Controlled, Add-On Trials in Adults with Partial Onset Seizures[a]

		TOPAMAX® Dosage (mg/day)		
Adverse Event	Placebo (N=216)	200 (N=45)	400 (N=68)	600-1,000 (N=414)
Fatigue	13	11	12	30
Nervousness	7	13	18	19
Difficulty with Concentration/ Attention	1	7	9	14
Confusion	4	9	10	14
Depression	6	9	7	13
Anorexia	4	4	6	12
Language problems	<1	2	9	10
Anxiety	6	2	3	10
Mood problems	2	0	6	9
Weight decrease	3	4	9	13

[a] Dose-response studies were not conducted for other adult indications or for pediatric indications.

Table 6: Incidence (%) of Treatment-Emergent Adverse Events in Placebo-Controlled, Add-On Trials in Pediatric Patients Ages 2-16 Years[a,b]
(Events That Occurred in at Least 1% of Topiramate-Treated Patients and Occurred More Frequently in Topiramate-Treated Than Placebo-Treated Patients)

Body System/ Adverse Event	Placebo (N=101)	Topiramate (N=98)
Body as a Whole – General Disorders		
Fatigue	5	16
Injury	13	14
Allergic Reaction	1	2
Back Pain	0	1
Pallor	0	1
Cardiovascular Disorders, General		
Hypertension	0	1
Central & Peripheral Nervous System Disorders		
Gait Abnormal	5	8
Ataxia	2	6
Hyperkinesia	4	5
Dizziness	2	4
Speech Disorders/Related Speech Problems	2	4
Hyporeflexia	0	2
Convulsions Grand Mal	0	1
Fecal Incontinence	0	1
Paresthesia	0	1
Gastro-Intestinal System Disorders		
Nausea	5	6
Saliva Increased	4	6
Constipation	4	5
Gastroenteritis	2	3
Dysphagia	0	1

Flatulence	0	1
Gastroesophageal Reflux	0	1
Glossitis	0	1
Gum Hyperplasia	0	1
Heart Rate and Rhythm Disorders		
Bradycardia	0	1
Metabolic and Nutritional Disorders		
Weight Decrease	1	9
Thirst	1	2
Hypoglycemia	0	1
Weight Increase	0	1
Platelet, Bleeding, & Clotting Disorders		
Purpura	4	8
Epistaxis	1	4
Hematoma	0	1
Prothrombin Increased	0	1
Thrombocytopenia	0	1
Psychiatric Disorders		
Somnolence	16	26
Anorexia	15	24
Nervousness	7	14
Personality Disorder (Behavior Problems)	9	11
Difficulty with Concentration/Attention	2	10
Aggressive Reaction	4	9
Insomnia	7	8
Difficulty with Memory NOS	0	5
Confusion	3	4
Psychomotor Slowing	2	3
Appetite Increased	0	1
Neurosis	0	1
Reproductive Disorders, Female		
Leukorrhoea	0	2
Resistance Mechanism Disorders		
Infection Viral	3	7
Respiratory System Disorders		
Pneumonia	1	5
Respiratory Disorder	0	1
Skin and Appendages Disorders		
Skin Disorder	2	3
Alopecia	1	2
Dermatitis	0	2
Hypertrichosis	1	2
Rash Erythematous	0	2
Eczema	0	1
Seborrhoea	0	1
Skin Discoloration	0	1
Urinary System Disorders		
Urinary Incontinence	2	4
Nocturia	0	1
Vision Disorders		
Eye Abnormality	1	2
Vision Abnormal	1	2
Diplopia	0	1
Lacrimation Abnormal	0	1
Myopia	0	1
White Cell and RES Disorders		
Leukopenia	0	2

[a] Patients in these add-on trials were receiving 1 to 2 concomitant antiepileptic drugs in addition to TOPAMAX® or placebo.

[b] Values represent the percentage of patients reporting a given adverse event. Patients may have reported more than one adverse event during the study and can be included in more than one adverse event category.

Other Adverse Events Observed
Other events that occurred in more than 1% of adults treated with 200 to 400 mg of topiramate in placebo-controlled trials but with equal or greater frequency in the placebo group were: headache, injury, anxiety, rash, pain, convulsions aggravated, coughing, fever, diarrhea, vomiting, muscle weakness, insomnia, personality disorder, dysmenorrhea, upper respiratory tract infection, and eye pain.

Other Adverse Events Observed During All Clinical Trials
Topiramate, initiated as adjunctive therapy, has been administered to 1,757 adults and 310 pediatric patients with epilepsy during all clinical studies. During these studies, all adverse events were recorded by the clinical investigators using terminology of their own choosing. To provide a meaningful estimate of the proportion of individuals having adverse events, similar types of events were grouped into a smaller number of standardized categories using modified WHOART dictionary terminology. The frequencies presented represent the proportion of patients who experienced an event of the type cited on at least one occasion while receiving topiramate. Reported events are included except those already listed in the previous table or text, those too general to be informative, and those not reasonably associated with the use of the drug.

Events are classified within body system categories and enumerated in order of decreasing frequency using the following definitions: *frequent* occurring in at least 1/100 patients; *infrequent* occurring in 1/100 to 1/1000 patients; *rare* occurring in fewer than 1/1000 patients.

Autonomic Nervous System Disorders: *Infrequent:* vasodilation.

Body as a Whole: *Frequent:* fever. *Infrequent:* syncope, abdomen enlarged. *Rare:* alcohol intolerance.

Cardiovascular Disorders, General: *Infrequent:* hypotension, postural hypotension.

Central & Peripheral Nervous System Disorders: *Frequent:* hypertonia. *Infrequent:* neuropathy, apraxia, hyperaesthesia, dyskinesia, dysphonia, scotoma, ptosis, dystonia, visual field defect, encephalopathy, upper motor neuron lesion, EEG abnormal. *Rare:* cerebellar syndrome, tongue paralysis.

Gastrointestinal System Disorders: *Frequent:* diarrhea, vomiting, hemorrhoids. *Infrequent:* stomatitis, melena, gastritis, tongue edema, esophagitis.

Hearing and Vestibular Disorders: *Frequent:* tinnitus.

Heart Rate and Rhythm Disorders: *Infrequent:* AV block, bradycardia.

Liver and Biliary System Disorders: *Infrequent:* SGPT increased, SGOT increased, gamma-GT increased.

Metabolic and Nutritional Disorders: *Frequent:* dehydration. *Infrequent:* hypokalemia, alkaline phosphatase increased, hypocalcemia, hyperlipemia, acidosis, hyperglycemia, hyperchloremia, xerophthalmia. *Rare:* diabetes mellitus, hypernatremia, hyponatremia, hypocholesterolemia, hypophosphatemia, creatinine increased.

Musculoskeletal System Disorders: *Frequent:* arthralgia, muscle weakness. *Infrequent:* arthrosis.

Myo-, Endo-, Pericardial & Valve Disorders: *Infrequent:* angina pectoris.

Neoplasms: *Infrequent:* thrombocythemia. *Rare:* polycythemia.

Platelet, Bleeding, and Clotting Disorders: *Infrequent:* gingival bleeding, pulmonary embolism.

Psychiatric Disorders: *Frequent:* impotence, hallucination, euphoria, psychosis. *Infrequent:* paranoid reaction, delusion, paranoia, delirium, abnormal dreaming, neurosis, libido increased, manic reaction, suicide attempt.

Red Blood Cell Disorders: *Frequent:* anemia. *Rare:* marrow depression, pancytopenia.

Reproductive Disorders, Male: *Infrequent:* ejaculation disorder, breast discharge.

Skin and Appendages Disorders: *Frequent:* acne, urticaria. *Infrequent:* photosensitivity reaction, sweating decreased, abnormal hair texture. *Rare:* chloasma.

Special Senses Other, Disorders: *Infrequent:* taste loss, parosmia.

Urinary System Disorders: *Frequent:* dysuria, renal calculus. *Infrequent:* urinary retention, face edema, renal pain, albuminuria, polyuria, oliguria.

Vascular (Extracardiac) Disorders: *Infrequent:* flushing, deep vein thrombosis, phlebitis. *Rare:* vasospasm.

Vision Disorders: *Frequent:* conjunctivitis. *Infrequent:* abnormal accommodation, photophobia, strabismus, mydriasis. *Rare:* iritis.

White Cell and Reticuloendothelial System Disorders: *Infrequent:* lymphadenopathy, eosinophilia, lymphopenia, granulocytopenia, lymphocytosis.

Postmarketing and Other Experience
In addition to the adverse experiences reported during clinical testing of TOPAMAX®, the following adverse experiences have been reported in patients receiving marketed TOPAMAX® from worldwide use since approval. These adverse experiences have not been listed above and data are insufficient to support an estimate of their incidence or to establish causation. The listing is alphabetized: hepatic failure, hepatitis, pancreatitis, and renal tubular acidosis.

DRUG ABUSE AND DEPENDENCE
The abuse and dependence potential of TOPAMAX® has not been evaluated in human studies.

OVERDOSAGE
In acute TOPAMAX® overdose, if the ingestion is recent, the stomach should be emptied immediately by lavage or by induction of emesis. Activated charcoal has not been shown to adsorb topiramate *in vitro*. Therefore, its use in overdosage is not recommended. Treatment should be appropriately supportive. Hemodialysis is an effective means of removing topiramate from the body. However, in the few cases of acute overdosage reported, hemodialysis has not been necessary.

DOSAGE AND ADMINISTRATION
TOPAMAX® has been shown to be effective in adults and pediatric patients ages 2-16 years with partial onset seizures or primary generalized tonic-clonic seizures, and in patients 2 years of age and older with seizures associated with Lennox-Gastaut syndrome. In the controlled add-on trials, no correlation has been demonstrated between trough plasma concentrations of topiramate and clinical efficacy. No evidence of tolerance has been demonstrated in humans. Doses above 400 mg/day (600, 800, or 1000 mg/day) have not been shown to improve responses in dose-response studies in adults with partial onset seizures.

It is not necessary to monitor topiramate plasma concentrations to optimize TOPAMAX® therapy. On occasion, the addition of TOPAMAX® to phenytoin may require an adjustment of the dose of phenytoin to achieve optimal clinical outcome. Addition or withdrawal of phenytoin and/or carbamazepine during adjunctive therapy with TOPAMAX® may require adjustment of the dose of TOPAMAX®. Because of the bitter taste, tablets should not be broken.

TOPAMAX® can be taken without regard to meals.

Adults (17 Years of Age and Over)
The recommended total daily dose of TOPAMAX® as adjunctive therapy is 400 mg/day in two divided doses. In studies of adults with partial onset seizures, a daily dose of 200 mg/day has inconsistent effects and is less effective than 400 mg/day. It is recommended that therapy be initiated at 25 - 50 mg/day followed by titration to an effective dose in increments of 25 - 50 mg/week. Titrating in increments of 25 mg/week may delay the time to reach an effective dose. Daily doses above 1,600 mg have not been studied.

In the study of primary generalized tonic-clonic seizures the initial titration rate was slower than in previous studies; the assigned dose was reached at the end of 8 weeks (see **CLINICAL STUDIES, Controlled Trials in Patients With Primary Generalized Tonic-Clonic Seizures**).

Pediatric Patients (Ages 2-16 Years) - Partial Seizures, Primary Generalized Tonic-Clonic Seizures, or Lennox-Gastaut Syndrome
The recommended total daily dose of TOPAMAX® (topiramate) as adjunctive therapy for patients with partial seizures, primary generalized tonic-clonic seizures, or seizures associated with Lennox-Gastaut Syndrome is approximately 5 to 9 mg/kg/day in two divided doses. Titration should begin at 25 mg (or less, based on a range of 1 to 3 mg/kg/day) nightly for the first week. The dosage should then be increased at 1- or 2-week intervals by increments of 1 to 3 mg/kg/day (administered in two divided doses), to achieve optimal clinical response. Dose titration should be guided by clinical outcome.

In the study of primary generalized tonic-clonic seizures the initial titration rate was slower than in previous studies; the assigned dose of 6 mg/kg/day was reached at the end of 8 weeks (see **CLINICAL STUDIES, Controlled Trials in Patients With Primary Generalized Tonic-Clonic Seizures**).

Administration of TOPAMAX® Sprinkle Capsules
TOPAMAX® (topiramate capsules) Sprinkle Capsules may be swallowed whole or may be administered by carefully opening the capsule and sprinkling the entire contents on a small amount (teaspoon) of soft food. This drug/food mixture should be swallowed immediately and not chewed. It should not be stored for future use.

Patients with Renal Impairment:
In renally impaired subjects (creatinine clearance less than 70 mL/min/1.73m^2), one half of the usual adult dose is recommended. Such patients will require a longer time to reach steady-state at each dose.

Patients Undergoing Hemodialysis:
Topiramate is cleared by hemodialysis at a rate that is 4 to 6 times greater than a normal individual. Accordingly, a prolonged period of dialysis may cause topiramate concentration to fall below that required to maintain an anti-seizure effect. To avoid rapid drops in topiramate plasma concentration during hemodialysis, a supplemental dose of topiramate may be required. The actual adjustment should take into account 1) the duration of dialysis period, 2) the clearance rate of the dialysis system being used, and 3) the effective renal clearance of topiramate in the patient being dialyzed.

Patients with Hepatic Disease:
In hepatically impaired patients topiramate plasma concentrations may be increased. The mechanism is not well understood.

HOW SUPPLIED
TOPAMAX® (topiramate) Tablets is available as debossed, coated, round tablets in the following strengths and colors:

25 mg white (coded "TOP" on one side; "25" on the other)

100 mg yellow (coded "TOPAMAX" on one side; "100" on the other)

200 mg salmon (coded "TOPAMAX" on one side; "200" on the other)

They are supplied as follows:

25 mg tablets - bottles of 60 count with desiccant (NDC 0045-0639-65)

100 mg tablets – bottles of 60 count with desiccant (NDC 0045-0641-65)

200 mg tablets – bottles of 60 count with desiccant (NDC 0045-0642-65)

TOPAMAX® (topiramate capsules) Sprinkle Capsules contain small, white to off white spheres. The gelatin capsules are white and clear.

They are marked as follows:

15 mg capsule with "TOP" and "15 mg" on the side

25 mg capsule with "TOP" and "25 mg" on the side

The capsules are supplied as follows:

15 mg capsules – bottles of 60 (NDC 0045-0647-65)

25 mg capsules – bottles of 60 (NDC 0045-0645-65)

TOPAMAX® (topiramate) Tablets should be stored in tightly-closed containers at controlled room temperature, (59 to 86°F, 15 to 30°C). Protect from moisture.

TOPAMAX® (topiramate capsules) Sprinkle Capsules should be stored in tightly-closed containers at or below 25°C (77°F). Protect from moisture.

TOPAMAX® (topiramate) and TOPAMAX® (topiramate capsules) are trademarks of Ortho-McNeil Pharmaceutical.

HOW TO TAKE
TOPAMAX® (topiramate capsules) SPRINKLE CAPSULES

A Guide for Patients and Their Caregivers

Your doctor has given you a prescription for TOPAMAX® (topiramate capsules) Sprinkle Capsules. Here are your instructions for taking this medication. Please read these instructions prior to use.

To Take With Food
You may sprinkle the contents of TOPAMAX® Sprinkle Capsules on a small amount (teaspoon) of soft food, such as applesauce, custard, ice cream, oatmeal, pudding, or yogurt.

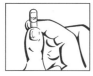

Hold the capsule upright so that you can read the word "TOP."

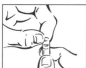

Carefully twist off the clear portion of the capsule. You may find it best to do this over the small portion of the food onto which you will be pouring the sprinkles.

Sprinkle all of the capsule's contents onto a spoonful of soft food, taking care to see that the entire prescribed dosage is sprinkled onto the food.

Be sure the patient swallows the entire spoonful of the sprinkle/food mixture immediately. Chewing should be avoided. It may be helpful to have the patient drink fluids immediately in order to make sure all of the mixture is swallowed.
IMPORTANT: Never store any sprinkle/food mixture for use at a later time.

To Take Without Food
TOPAMAX® Sprinkle Capsules may also be swallowed as whole capsules.

For more information about TOPAMAX® Sprinkle Capsules, ask your doctor or pharmacist.

ORTHO-McNEIL

OMP DIVISION
ORTHO-McNEIL PHARMACEUTICAL, INC.
Raritan, NJ 08869
© OMP 1999   Revised September 2001   7517102

NOTES

NOTES